Clinical Thinking

WITHDRAWN

2 6 MAR 2023

Clinical Thinking

Evidence, Communication and Decision-Making

Chris Del Mar
Bond University, Queensland, Australia

Jenny Doust
University of Queensland, Queensland, Australia

Paul Glasziou
University of Oxford, Oxford, UK

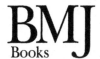

Blackwell
Publishing

Published by Blackwell Publishing Ltd
BMJ Books is an imprint of the BMJ Publishing Group Limited, used under licence

Blackwell Publishing Inc., 350 Main Street, Malden, Massachusetts 02148-5020, USA
Blackwell Publishing Ltd, 9600 Garsington Road, Oxford OX4 2DQ, UK
Blackwell Publishing Asia Pty Ltd, 550 Swanston Street, Carlton, Victoria 3053, Australia

First published 2006

4   2008

Library of Congress Cataloging-in-Publication Data

Del Mar, Chris.
    Clinical thinking : evidence, communication and decision-making / Chris Del Mar,
Jenny Doust, Paul Glasziou.
    p. ; cm.
    Includes bibliographical references
    ISBN: 978-0-7279-1741-6
1. Clinical medicine–Decision making.   2. Evidence-based medicine.
    [DNLM: 1. Patient Care Management–methods.   2. Communication.
3. Decision Making.   4. Diagnostic Techniques and Procedures.   5. Evidence-Based
Medicine–methods.   6. Problem Solving. W 84.7 D359c 2006]   I. Doust, Jenny.
II. Glasziou, Paul, 1954-   III. Title.

    R723.5.D45 2006
    616–dc22

                                                                    2005037642

A catalogue record for this title is available from the British Library

Set in 9.5/12pt Meridien by TechBooks, India

Commissioning Editor: Mary Banks
Editorial Assistant: Victoria Pittman
Development Editor: Elisabeth Dodds
Production Controller: Kate Charman

For further information on Blackwell Publishing, visit our website:
www.blackwellpublishing.com

The publisher's policy is to use permanent paper from mills that operate a sustainable
forestry policy, and which has been manufactured from pulp processed using acid-free
and elementary chlorine-free practices. Furthermore, the publisher ensures that the text
paper and cover board used have met acceptable environmental accreditation standards.

Contents

Foreword

Every experienced doctor appreciates – and every newly-qualified doctor quickly discovers – that knowing the facts is not the same as knowing what to do. Diseases don't conform to the textbook versions. Patients can be idiosyncratic and sometimes irrational. So can doctors. Research evidence is often inconsistent, and even the most up-to-date paper is never the last word. The so-called information explosion can confuse as easily as it can illuminate. Every protocol, guideline and code of good practice immediately reminds the practising clinician of a hundred exceptions.

The hallmark of the trustworthy doctor – many would say it is a defining characteristic of a true professional – is the ability to make judgements in the face of uncertainty. Doctors have to be good at interpreting, at prioritising, at making compromises, at seeing what matters amid a welter of complication, and at sometimes insisting that what seems right in theory would be damaging in the flesh. Faced with such a complex task, it is tempting to take refuge in a number of easy but flawed positions. 'I will only ever do what I can justify with evidence' is one such. 'I'll just do what I always do, or what my teachers always did' is another. But the first soon leads to paralysis, the second to dangerous sloppiness. Sound clinical thinking, and the professional judgement that flows from it, is neither slavishly obedient to any rule nor recklessly disregarding of the best available information.

The question for doctors at every stage of their careers is how their thinking skills are to be acquired, developed, honed, maintained, and protected against inertia and atrophy. Surfing the exponential wave of new knowledge is necessary, but not sufficient. Preserving one's fascination with human nature in its many manifestations through literature, the arts and humanities is helpful, desirable, but not – for some specialities at least – essential. The necessary complement to both these is to cultivate the habit of critical reflection upon one's own practice, conducted with genuine curiosity and humility. Self-reflection is another defining characteristic of a true professional, and that is what this book embodies. To read it is to learn the value of thinking about how one thinks. The reader will benefit, but his or her patients will do so in greater measure. Patients deserve to have doctors who not only know their stuff but also know how to apply that knowledge to the human predicaments that daily confront them.

Roger Neighbour MA DSc FRCP PRCGP
President, Royal College of General Practitioners
Bedmond, December 2005

Preface: what this book is about

This book is designed to help people understand the clinical thinking needed to practice successfully.

It is based on the simple notion that there are two sorts of learning that we need for practice: knowledge and skills (of the diagnosis and management of diseases and associated symptoms), and the ability to synthesise this information into clinical decisions. The knowledge and skills can be further subdivided into *background* information (the basic information, made up of anatomy, biochemistry, physiology, psychology, pathology and so on) needed to understand the principles of caring for sick people, and the *foreground* information (the research which best guides management).

Practicing medicine is not just about recalling facts, however. It is about being able to process the facts in order to make *choices*. All of clinical work can be thought of as decisions, even such hands-on skill-based activities such as surgery. Of course, the first set of learning enables one to decide what the choices are. But having assembled the necessary information, how does one go about deciding what actually to *do*?

The major revolution in *foreground* information has been the rising star of evidence-based practice (EBP), or evidence-based medicine (EBM). This has changed the way we think of knowledge: no longer the static stuff that can be hauled out of books or stuffed into the heads of medical students and registrars, but something dynamic that we should be pulling down electronically, often, and not even bothering to remember because it will be out of date by the time we have committed it to memory. We all three are very interested in EBP. But that is not the subject of this little book. Rather we wrote this to help set out (as much as anything for our own minds!) some of the cognitive processes that we think make it easier to apply the knowledge and skills into clinical practice. We three decided, while enjoying the brainstorming that went into preparing for the book, that we wished something like it had been written for us when we were students and registrars.

What we have done in this book is to gather together what is known about the art and the science of how we use the facts of medicine to solve the problems we face as clinicians. Some of the science is counter-intuitive. This is what makes it so fascinating. We have included some of the items that we find helpful or unexpected, and tried to synthesise them into a story. Hopefully you too will find that this is not only helpful, but also makes clinical practice even more fun. Where evidence for some of the more outrageous claims exists

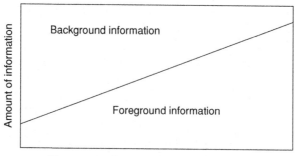

Time: maturation as a clinician →

Figure Different types of information needed for successful clinical practice. Adapted from Sackett et al.[1]

we have quoted it. But on the whole this book is not so much an academic exercise as a handbook. Hopefully, it will help us all to be better clinicians. We hope you find it so.

The way the book is written is to set out the framework of the thinking in chapters. We often illustrate the principles with a 'case' (many from our own practices) to help show how they might be applied, and then at the end of each section we show how they could be applied into clinical practice by explaining them to the 'patient' as a dialogue.

Who are we? We are academic general practitioners who met up in Queensland. We all worked in the same clinical general practice while we worked together in academia, before spreading out. We did a certain amount of sitting around, drinking green tea and thinking about this book. One consequence of our background is that our examples are firmly based on primary care. For this we make no apology. We think that if one can get clinical thinking to be useful in general practice, that seat of the greatest unknown, least differentiated disease, then it is likely to be useful almost anywhere in clinical practice.

We dedicate the book to patients, for whom we hope this will make a difference, reduce their suffering, and help their doctors manage their illnesses better.

Chris Del Mar
Jenny Doust
Paul Glasziou

CHAPTER 1

Principles of clinical problem solving

Doctors constantly make decisions. It may not always feel like this. In fact, if we have been in practice for a while, it can begin to feel as if much of our practice is routine. This is because 'when things are proceeding normally, experts don't solve problems and don't make decisions: they do what normally works'.[2]

Part of becoming a competent doctor is learning the vast number of facts necessary to practice medicine. The more important part of our learning is to model the decision-making behaviour of more experienced clinicians, learning the routines that they use to collect and process the facts of each new case and thereby learn to make the sort of decisions that we all need to make as clinicians (see Box 1.1).

Our clinical training gives us the context and the experience to process the information of each new patient and to map it against our store of memorised facts. The way that we listen to and recount the stories of our patients becomes ritualised, with strict rules like a Greek chorus. The textbook facts that we have learnt begin to attach themselves to experience, to the stories of our patients and to our own experience of working in health care. We now know that clinical knowledge is mostly stored in memory as stories or templates, and not as collections of abstracted facts.[3] As we gain clinical experience, we are gradually able to use the details that we see and hear with better discrimination and with time we come to make decisions more or less intuitively, and may even find it difficult to explain the intermediate steps in our clinical reasoning (Box 1.2).

Box 1.1 Examples of Typical Clinical Decisions

- Should I do a test? Which test should I do?
- Could I be missing a diagnosis? Should I be investigating this patient further?
- Which of the available drugs should I prescribe? Would the patient be better without further medication?
- Is it alright to divide this structure during the operation – am I sure it is a vein and not a nerve...?
- Should I ask the patient to come back? When? How often?

> **Box 1.2 Characteristics of Novice, Competent and Expert Practitioners[4]**
>
> *The novice practitioner is characterised by:*
> Rigid adherence to taught rules or plans
> Little situational perception
> No discretionary judgment
>
> *The competent practitioner:*
> Is able to cope with 'crowdedness' and pressure
> Sees actions partly in terms of long-term goals or a wider conceptual framework
> Follows standardised and routinised procedures
>
> *The expert practitioner:*
> No longer relies explicitly on rules, guidelines and maxims
> Has an intuitive grasp of situations based on deep, tacit understanding
> Uses analytic approaches only in novel situations or when problems occur

Because of our training and experience, we are able to practice medicine without considering in great detail how we come to make clinical decisions. Many expert and highly competent clinicians have not studied the principles outlined in this book. We believe, however, that learning the principles of clinical problem solving is important in order to provide the best possible care for our patients, and that understanding these principles will be increasingly important for medical care in the future.

Firstly, understanding the methods for clinical problem solving is important when a problem arises where we do not have a routine or practiced approach. By its nature, this happens more frequently in general practice than in any other area of medicine. It is probably no accident that the three authors of this book, and many authors who write in this area, come from general practice backgrounds. But being able to deal with new and complex problems and being able to manage uncertainty is important in all areas of clinical medicine. Being able to understand the principles of clinical problem solving is particularly important when we are relatively junior and have not yet developed enough clinical experience to act more intuitively.

Secondly, understanding these principles gives us a framework for incorporating both new evidence and the values of our patients into our clinical decisions. Evidence-based medicine is described as 'the integration of best research evidence with clinical expertise and patient values'[1], but it is not always clear to clinicians how this integration might occur. Two changes make it imperative to find methods for such integration. The first is the rate at which new medical knowledge is advancing. The second is the greater desire for patients to participate in decisions about their own health care. As another leader of the evidence-based medicine movement described it: 'medicine is indeed in the middle of an intellectual revolution. Methods of reasoning and problem solving that might have worked well in the past are not sufficient to handle today's problems.'[5] The framework outlined in this book shows how the integration between clinical expertise, research evidence and patient values can begin to occur.

Thirdly, there are times when we can predict that intuitive or routine decision making might fail. Being aware of the potential cognitive biases in our routine thinking can help us to be better and safer doctors.

Finally, we have found that learning and thinking about the principles of clinical problem solving has improved our understanding of what we are doing as clinicians. All three of us have found that understanding these principles makes our clinical work more fun.

The framework for clinical problem solving

Studies of naturalistic decision making have shown that experts making critical decisions, such as fire commanders in charge of units fighting large fires, are often unaware of making any decisions.[6] This is even though they clearly have to make decisions such as the need for extra units, when to withdraw firefighters from a situation and so on. When asked to explain their decision-making process, the fire commanders will usually insist that they do not make decisions and that it is obvious what to do in any given situation. After analysis of how they actually made critical decisions, it seems that experts use their experience to match each new situation to a prototype, and to use this prototype to decide on a course of action. They may recognise that they need to collect more data to clarify a situation or to re-evaluate a situation if conditions change over time, but at each point they are trying to match the situation to a prototype. The main elements of the recognition primed decision-making model are shown in Figure 1.1. This model appears to be very consistent with what we know about how expert clinicians make decisions in medicine (Box 1.3).[7] For example, when a patient is admitted with a myocardial infarction, it is important to decide quickly whether a patient should have thrombolytic therapy or not. There are many factors that could determine this choice, but it has been shown, in fact, that doctors use only a few of these features to make the decision. Doctors are often better than clinical algorithms or decision support systems could be at determining when the clinical pattern does not fit. For example, a case report in *The Lancet* describes a patient who presented with chest pain and ST segment elevation in the anterior leads.[8] The medical team was preparing to give the patient thrombolytic therapy, when the patient remarked that he could not move or feel his legs. Recognising that this did not fit the clinical pattern of myocardial infarction, the team investigated further. A CT of the patient's chest and abdomen showed a thoracic aortic dissection.

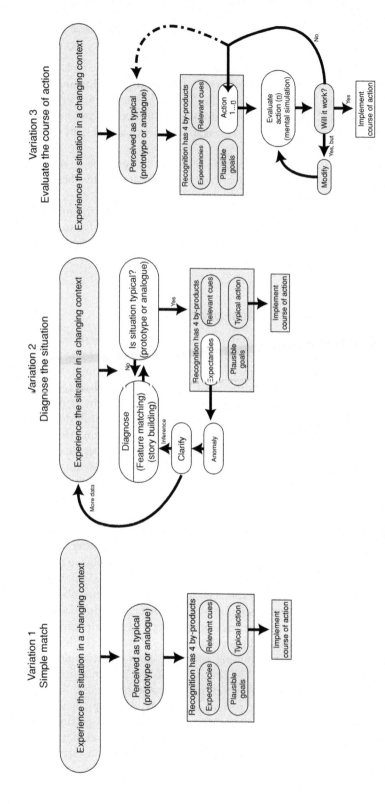

Figure 1.1 Recognition primed decision model.[6]

4

Box 1.3 The Case of a 28-Year-Old Man With a Fever and a Sore Bottom

During training as a general practice registrar, one of us saw a patient with these symptoms. I checked him carefully, but could find no cause for the fever (38.5°C). A *per rectum* examination revealed nothing specific (except it slightly exacerbated the rectal pain he had).

I told him I couldn't find the cause for the fever, and that it was probably an early virus infection (despite the lack of respiratory symptoms). I couldn't explain the rectal pain, but was reassured by the essentially normal examination. I suggested he should return if things got any worse.

But later that day, talking the case over with a more experienced general practitioner, he suggested ischio-rectal abscess. I had not thought of that. I rang the clinic, had the patient brought back, and referred him to hospital for investigation. It was as suspected, and he had a drainage operation later.

Later I wondered about the case. How was it the experienced GP had got this right? There were probably several factors. My obvious concern about the case (something was clearly not right: this is called 'dissonance from the expected'); the pattern that he recognised immediately; the diagnosis he had seen before; and the method of not 'missing' things – making sure that diagnoses that matter are checked out carefully.

An alternative model of decision making is based on rational choice strategies (see Box 1.4).[9] Using this approach, we can think of health care decisions as consisting of three major steps, with each major step having three minor steps (Pro-Act-Ive). We will lay out the steps in sequence (see Box 1.5), but it is important to keep in mind that the steps need not occur sequentially. Sometimes the choice in a decision becomes clear before all the steps have been taken; at other times, a later step will make it necessary to go back and repeat an earlier step in an iterative process. Also, it is important to recognise that doctors only use this approach with novel or complex problems. In situations where they are familiar with the problem and its diagnosis and treatment, they will act according to their experience and usually will not be aware of making decisions in an explicit sense at all.

Box 1.4 Decision–Making Theory

Many of the principles described here are based on medical adaptations[8] of rational decision-making theory.[9] Decision theory was originally developed to explain how economic organisations make decisions.[10]

Box 1.5 The Components of Decision Making: Pro-Act-Ive

	Mnemonic	Element	Tasks
Sorting out the problem	P	Problem	Define it. How does the diagnosis affect health?
	R	Reframe the problem	From multiple perspectives: think of everyone's, now and in the future
	O	Objectives	What is the best outcome we could achieve? Take into consideration other health influences and diagnoses
Action	A	Alternatives	List these, collapsing them into basic options: (e.g., treat; wait-and-see; *or* test)
	C	Consequences	Imagine the outcome of each alternative – especially nothing!
	T	Trade-offs	Often (but not always) it is worth talking treatment risks (e.g., surgery) for long-term benefits
Integration	I	Integration of	When pulling it all together for a decision, remember the patient
	V	Values	may have unexpected values.
	E	Exploration	These cannot be assumed and need to be explored with the patient

The Pro-Act-Ive approach to decision making in health care

Decision making involves a lot of steps. The Pro-Act-Ive mnemonic helps avoid missing any (see Box 1.5).

PRO – defining the problem and the objectives

P = defining the problem

The first step in any decision is to define the problem. In health care, this is not just deciding on the diagnosis. It means defining how the diagnosis or health care problem affects the patient.

For example, type II diabetes is not generally a problem for patients immediately (which is why so many people are unaware that they have the disorder). It is a problem because of the potential micro-vascular and macro-vascular complications that can occur over time.

We need to consider carefully how the diagnosis of a medical condition impacts on the life of the patient.

R = reframe the problem from multiple perspectives

When first thinking through a clinical problem, we need to think as broadly as possible. Many problems and the actions taken to address them can have unexpected consequences. Trying to think through the problem from as many perspectives as possible can help to ensure we have considered as many possible consequences as possible. Who is affected by the problem is also important. Any health care problem is likely to affect not only the patient, but also their family and their community.

O — focus on the objectives

After carefully considering the problem and its possible consequences, we can define the objectives that we are trying to achieve.

While managing a patient with type 2 diabetes, we may decide to focus on minimising the risk of long-term complications, but there may be multiple other objectives. How important is it to avoid the side effects or complications from the treatment? Are there different objectives in the short- and the long-term? How will the patient's life expectancy and other health problems impact on these objectives?

The patient and the clinician need to agree on the objectives. It is clear that doctors often fail in this area.

Doctors are unable to predict which patients are requesting a script for an antibiotic when presenting with a diarrhoea.[11]

Clinicians must never assume that they know or understand the objectives of the patient or that all patients will have similar objectives. Some clinical scenarios can make the different values and objectives of patients with the same disease very stark.

Some patients with cancer will choose any treatment that gives them a greater chance of survival, no matter what the side effects. Others will prefer a shorter life span, but with greater quality of life.

As we will discuss in the next chapter, being able to come to a shared agreement on the objectives of management is one of the most important tasks in a consultation. Sometimes we will have intermediate markers that help us guide treatment.

In managing diabetes an intermediate objective may be to normalise the HbA1c.

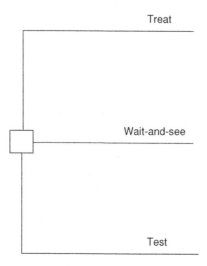

Treat

Wait-and-see

Test

Figure 1.2 Generic decision tree.

However, we should not forget that this is an intermediate marker (a biological endpoint that has little effect on the patient's quality of life) and is useful only because it relates to our more fundamental objectives of trying to reduce the risk of long-term complications.

Act – determining the alternatives, consequences and trade-offs

A = consider all relevant alternatives

Once we have thought through the problem and the possible objectives, we need to consider all the potentially relevant alternatives. Sometimes there can be many complex and branching alternatives. We might want to collapse the many alternatives into some generic decisions to begin with (see Figure 1.2). Many clinical decisions can fit the generic model of: treat, wait and see and obtain more information (such as further tests).[8]

It is especially important to consider the wait-and-see alternative. Active intervention is not always necessary, or may not be the best option to fix a problem (as we will see in Chapter 6).

C = consider the consequences of each alternative and estimate the chances

To choose between several alternative courses of action, we need to consider the potential consequences of each alternative. This is the point that we begin to consider the evidence. Being able to find the best possible evidence on the potential benefits and harms of treatment can be critical to a decision.

> For example, if we are considering the management of a patient who has recently been diagnosed with type 2 diabetes, we have several possible management choices. We need to consider, for example, what is likely to happen to the patient if we begin with lifestyle interventions

such as diet and exercise? What is likely to happen if we begin with a sulphonylurea? Or a biguanide? What would happen if we did nothing? Could we combine some of these alternatives? How will each of these alternatives affect the patient's objectives? Are there other potential consequences not thought of in the context of the original problem, such as the patient's sense of empowerment? What are the potential costs to the patient and to the society of each action? Are there any potential harms?

T = identify and estimate the trade-offs
There can be many different consequences for each alternative course of action.

In the diabetes example, one alternative is better for some consequences (diet and lifestyle are cheaper and have other health benefits), while another alternative will be better for other areas (biguanides may normalise the blood sugar levels more quickly and help with weight loss).

We need to consider the potential trade-offs for the consequences of each alternative. Again, the patient needs to be central to this discussion. Different patients can place very different values on the potential consequences of each alternative.

Consider a patient who has suffered a transient ischaemic attack (TIA) and is found to have a carotid artery stenosis. The patient is at risk of a further TIA or even a stroke. But the surgery to correct the stenosis also has a risk of stroke or death. Is the patient willing to take a short-term increased risk of mortality against a better long-term prognosis?

Ive – integration and exploration

I = integrate the evidence and the values
Once we are clear about the possible alternatives, the potential consequences of the alternatives and the values we place on these consequences, we need to integrate this information so that we can make a decision. The best option may be obvious. In fact, laying out the options may make this apparent and further consideration unnecessary. At other times the decision will be more complex with important consequences developing from competing alternatives. It may be necessary to consider all or some of the above steps more closely. Sometimes the decision may be primarily probability driven (affected by the probability of the potential risks and benefits); at other times, it will be primarily value-driven (affected by the values of the patient) or it may be both.

There has been an ongoing debate whether patients with non-ST elevated myocardial infarction benefit most from an interventional approach (investigate all patients and provide revascularisation wherever possible), or a conservative approach (only investigate and revascularise with continued symptoms).

It appears that the decision depends both on the probability of benefit (which is related to the underlying risk of the patient) and the values of the patient (there is some early mortality risk but a longer-term increased chance of survival).[12]

V = optimise the expected value

Now that we have integrated all the available information, we can choose the alternative that has the consequences that best meet our overall objectives.

At this point, it is worthwhile reconsidering the dictum ascribed to Hippocrates: 'first, do no harm'. If it was truly our objective as clinicians to do no harm, we would be unable to instigate anything other than a few lifesaving medical or surgical treatments (maybe antivenene for snake bite). Every treatment has potential risks. The benefits of treatment are highly variable, as is the natural history of the disease.

Many patients with type 2 diabetes will suffer no health consequences as a result of their disease. Others will suffer severe complications, including renal disease, myocardial infarction and death.

We are only able to predict the potential benefits for groups of patients, not for the individual patient in front of us. As doctors, we are constantly trying to balance the potential benefits and risks of alternative treatment (including no active treatment) and trying to maximise the overall (net) benefits.

Not infrequently, our patients will have an entirely different and unexpected perception of the potential risks and benefits of treatment.

Some patients refuse interventions that appear to us to carry little risk (such as immunisation or X-rays), because of their view of the balance of risks and benefits.

We often need to know about them (see Chapter 2 on Communication).

E = explore the assumptions and evaluate uncertainty

There may be uncertainty that affects our ability to make a decision, particularly about the benefits of treatment or the values that our patients might place on the consequences. We may want to test how sensitive our final decision is by considering what our decision would be if we changed these values. Is one alternative clearly better? Or is it a toss-up (such as the management of NSTEMI discussed above)? If a decision is very sensitive to the size of the treatment benefit, we might want to 'invest' more time and effort in obtaining more accurate estimates of the size of the benefit for patients or for a stratified group of patients. For example, one strategy in the management of NSTEMI may be to identify those patients who are most at risk of further complications and who are therefore most likely to benefit from the more interventional strategy.

Recognition primed decision making versus rational decision making

To carry out each of the steps outlined in the Pro-Act-Ive model is obviously complex. Assembling all the information and constructing and analysing a decision analysis for a health care decision can be months of work. It is impractical to complete each of these steps to make a decision in a busy clinical environment. It is also not in line with what we know about how doctors make decisions in real life. In real life, we act much more in line with the recognition primed decision-making model, matching each new clinical situation to our past experience (in the form of stories and scripts) and act in accordance with what we know from our training and experience to do in that situation.

The rational decision-making model is still useful, however. It makes our decision-making process more explicit. When there is uncertainty about management or new information is available, we may want to invest the time (generally as a professional group) to develop and investigate the information, for example by writing a clinical guideline. The best form of these guidelines incorporates all the current evidence and explicitly states the potential harms and benefits of treatments. What guidelines cannot do, however, is to incorporate all the factors that may be important to a patient in making a decision, such as their own values and objectives.

Understanding the principles of the rational decision-making model is also helpful in everyday clinical decision making. Being aware of the alternatives, the potential consequences and the possible harms and benefits of our actions is enough to make us more aware and thoughtful clinicians. We do not need to be able to do a complete decision analysis to make these principles useful. Ensuring that we confirm the objectives and the values of our patients makes our consultations more 'patient centred'. Being able to systematically think through these principles allows us to explicitly consider the consequences of our clinical decisions, to incorporate the evidence on the potential harms and benefits and to incorporate the values of our patients into the decision-making process. It explains the place of clinical evidence in the decision-making process.

Summary

In this book, we will describe the general principles of clinical problem solving as they apply to all types of clinical decisions: diagnosis, prognosis, management, monitoring patients and so forth. We will describe both what is known about how doctors make such decisions, and ways that we believe can help doctors to improve their clinical problem solving. Our hope is that with greater understanding of these principles, doctors will be able to provide both safer and more patient-centred care.

CHAPTER 2

Communication in clinical care

Words are, of course, the most powerful drug used by mankind.

Rudyard Kipling

We have seen how every clinical decision needs exploration of patient values. There is a lot more important two-way traffic of information as well.

Doctor: *'Good morning Mr Smith. What can I do for you today?'*

Many clinicians assume they are good at communicating. Often they are not. It seems to be such a non-technical part of clinical work that few ever consider that they might be able to do it better. Yet, in surveys of the community that ask what people see as major deficiencies in their doctors, inadequate communicating features large.[13] Clinicians are often horrified when patients express dissatisfaction with their care, make a complaint or sue them. The most common cause is some sort of failure in communication. It is important for other reasons too: good communication improves patient outcomes.[14]

Good communication improves patient outcomes

Many models of communication have been constructed. Most are designed to help doctors improve the way they talk with and listen to their patients. Some models have improved the way we work, although their evaluation is often (surprisingly) inadequate. That is, most models are more theoretical than empirical. Nevertheless, they have shaped the way we think about communicating with patients.

Beginnings: 'take a full history . . . '

The traditional model of communicating with patients is what many doctors were taught at medical school. It is still the 'first' model students are taught in many medical programs today (see Box 2.1).

The process is straightforward. It is often ritualised to help novices avoid missing important elements. The patient 'presents' a clinical problem (*the presenting complaint*). The clinician asks questions to find out what the patient is experiencing in relation to this problem (*symptoms*). These questions often

Box 2.1 Where the History Sits Within a Traditional Doctor–Patient Consultation

- Presenting complaint
- History of the presenting complaint
- Review of the systems
- Examination
- Diagnosis
- Special tests
- Treatment

follow a format (for example, asking about pain usually requires asking specific questions (see Box 2.2).

This order of the elements in the consultation is not rigid. In emergencies treatment comes before anything else, certainly a specific diagnosis.

Sometimes the history is partly conducted during the examination.

'... Have you had any pain here...?'

One reassuring action is to provide a running commentary to the patient during the examination to provide reassurance or, at least, feedback.

'... Now I am just feeling on this side to see if the liver is enlarged, no, that feels quite normal, and nice and soft which is normal too, so let's just check that the spleen isn't enlarged on the other side here...'

This can forewarn the patient of what you will do. It also lets them know what you have (and have not!) found.

Clinicians are now often taught to provide such commentaries during vaginal speculum examinations, but it is useful in *any* examination, or even near-patient testing (such as ECGs or urine tests).

Box 2.2 Typical Questions About Pain

- Previous episodes
- Position – where it starts
- Radiation – where it moves to
- Timing – duration and whether constant, colicky, continuous or episodic, etc.
- Severity
- Associated symptoms
- Factors that appear to worsen it or relieve it
- Precipitating events
- Other questions etc.

Table 2.1 Different cognitive models used to arrive at a diagnosis.

Type of cognitive process	Characteristics	Examples
Full systematic history and examination	Slow: exhaustive – minimises the forgetting of important possibilities	
Hypothetico-deductive reasoning	Faster: concentrates the gathering of information into provisional diagnoses generated very early, raising new possibilities readily	Surgeon's diagnosis of acute abdominal pain
Pattern recognition	Fastest: relies on experience. Less helpful for problems not encountered before, or remembered	Spot diagnosis of mumps

Different cognitive models used for diagnosis are explored in greater depth in Chapter 4.

The first part of the traditional consultation is often called *the history of the presenting complaint*. Other questions of a more general nature about the patient's health follow, perhaps unrelated initially to the presenting problem (*review of systems*). This all constitutes the patient's narrative (*the history*).

Taking a history is the major part of a consultation process. Next follows the clinical examination, during which more information about the patient is gathered. Finally, clinicians may order investigations to provide yet more information (some can be undertaken immediately – such as a urine dipstick test, or ECG – and others cannot yield a result for days or longer, including blood tests and X-rays). At some stage the clinician develops some diagnostic possibilities. These hypotheses are called the *differential diagnosis*, a list. To refine the list more questions might be asked, more examination undertaken or more tests ordered. Out of the differential diagnosis comes the *provisional diagnosis* (or, when things are unclear, *diagnoses*). This forms the basis of management. Sometimes the provisional diagnosis has to be revised because the course of the illness, or its response to treatment, behaves unexpectedly.

Novices working at developing these skills often treat this whole thing as a puzzle. Having amassed a lot of information, they then sit down to synthesise diagnostic answers. What is often astonishing to them is the speed at which experienced clinicians arrive at a provisional diagnosis. It is clear that experienced doctors work on different cognitive models (see Chapter 4 on Diagnosis and Table 2.1).

Experienced clinicians often use all methods of arriving at a diagnosis, depending on their familiarity with the clinical problem. Difficult and unfamiliar problems require the slower full systematic history and examination methods, while the familiar well-encountered problems are quickly diagnosed with pattern recognition.

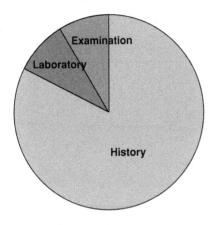

Figure 2.1 Contributions of history, examination and laboratory investigations of 80 different patients' diagnoses in a hospital internist outpatient clinic.[15]

Novices also soon discover that more information is derived from the *history* than the *examination* (see Figure 2.1).

It is often worth spending disproportionately more time talking than prodding or testing.[15] Within the *history* the *review of systems* seems to be especially unproductive, and few experienced clinicians make use of this fishing expedition.[16]

Very often *investigations* are used to *confirm* or *exclude* diagnoses (see Chapter 4 on Diagnosis).

This practical system (Box 2.1) is very useful for helping clinicians find a label to direct management. But there is a drawback: patients often find the process de-humanising. They do not feel 'listened to', nor that the things that are important to them register with the doctor.

The quality of communication

The literature focussing on the quality of communication is surprisingly short. One key study consisted of carefully listening to audiotapes of primary care consultations in the 1970s.[17] Some consultations were clearly much better than others.

A particular concern is that doctors tend to override their patients, interrupting their flow and re-directing the agenda. In less than half of the consultations did patients get their important concerns addressed.[18,19] So, although doctors might feel they arrive at the correct diagnosis, the patient may feel their real problems or concerns remain unexpressed. Good medicine should always include good communication.

This begs the question of how consultation communication quality might be measured. One obvious way is to measure *patient satisfaction*. This has become caught up with the notion of patients as consumers, and marks a shift in attitude away from doctors as all-knowing beneficent professionals. What are

Table 2.2 Tasks of the consultation (modified from Pendleton).[20]

Task	What this means
1	Define the reasons for the patient's attendance: Nature and history of the problems. Their aetiology. The patient's ideas, concerns and expectations. The effects of the problems.
2	Consider other problems: Continuing problems. At-risk factors.
3	Achieve a shared understanding of problems.
4	Involve patients in choosing and implementing management.
5	Encourage the taking of responsibility for health.
6	Use time and resources appropriately.
7	Establish or maintain a relationship with the patient that helps to achieve these tasks.

the factors important in leading to successful consultations, and those to less successful ones?

Communication obligations and responsibilities: 'tasks of the consultation'

One line of inquiry suggested that there were several *tasks* that are important (see Table 2.2).[20]

The most important of these was to not take at face value what patients present to the doctor. Even if the patient has specific concerns, they may not be stated directly, and sometimes we need to dig a little to find the *real* problem, which is deeper. Understanding these issues might be essential to helping effectively (see Box 2.3).

Understanding why the patient has come: a clinical example

Mukesh Habib is a young man with chest pain. He was seen at the hospital Emergency Department last week. The doctor there took a history

Box 2.3 Balancing Consumerism and Paternalism

		Clinician control	
		Low	*High*
Patient control	*Low*	(Good for no-one)	Paternalism
	High	Consumerism	Mutual

Box 2.4 Example of 'Agendas Model'

Presenting complaint	Doctor's agenda	Patient's agenda (*example*)
Pain in chest	1 'Exclude myocardial infarction.' 2 'Check there are no other medical problems.' 3 'Check other preventive activities.'	1 'Tell me I am not going to die.' 2 'Do the right tests (whatever they are).' 3 'Be explicit about pulmonary embolus . . .'

and examined him. History, examination and tests (including ECG and cardiac enzyme assay) suggested myocardial infarction was very unlikely.

But Mukesh remains very anxious. He re-presents to the Emergency Department, is reviewed and is reassured again. He goes to his primary care doctor, who discovers that he is worried about pulmonary embolus: he witnessed a fellow work-mate die of it recently.

This diagnosis is also (on the same clinical basis) very unlikely, and this was communicated effectively to the patient. He was now satisfied, and the pain no longer frightened him. Knowing the doctor had thought of what was worrying him was re-assuring.

This task gives clinicians the responsibility of ensuring they know *why* the patient is concerned. (See Box 2.4 to see a worked example using a model to disentangle the issues.)

There are other clinical responsibilities of the consultation that go beyond communication. Some of the most useful models are the simplest (see Table 2.3).

In the 'potentials for optimal care' model, the several tasks are lumped into just four (easier to remember!). The authors of this model suggest gluing a card with this Table at head height just behind the patient's chair for easy

Table 2.3 The 'potentials for optimal care' model.[21]

Why did the patient come?	What other medical problems can be dealt with?
A	B
C	D
Can health promotion or disease prevention be offered?	Can the patient be made more self-sufficient?

reference.[21] In the clinical examples we have discussed so far, the optimal care involves focussing on the top left quadrant (Table 2.3 quadrant A).

But the other quadrants are also important:

Every consultation is an opportunity to address other important health problems already diagnosed. These need to be thought of as background to the acute problem that the patient might draw to your attention (Table 2.3 quadrant B).

'Mukesh, let me just check up what happened to that funny rash you had last year. Did the ointment I gave you resolve it satisfactorily?'

And of course the principle of *opportunistic prevention* (see Chapter 8 on Screening, Health promotion and Prevention) requires one to think of some useful health promotion or disease prevention activity that might be brought up at every consultation, the 'exceptional potential' for doing so (Table 2.3 quadrant C). We discuss this in more detail in Chapter 8 on Screening.

'Remind me Mukesh, you're not a smoker, are you? Good. Now then let me just check your blood pressure because we don't have a reading here for several years. . .'

Finally, it is also worth checking off in one's mind that both doctor and patient have a clear idea what needs to happen with respect to meeting again (Table 2.3 quadrant D).

'Good. That's everything then. You've got some paracetamol* at home for the pain which neither of us are worried about now, and we don't need to see you again unless the pain gets worse or there's something new. OK. Is there anything else?'

One problem with the development of these models was the apparent conflict between patient autonomy ('consumerism', with its attendant danger of inappropriate health spending), and clinician's paternalism (with its insufficient recognition of patients' values and needs) (See Box 2.3).

One way of achieving this is the notion of 'agendas': the clinician has one, and so does the patient (and perhaps also important others, such as family members).[22] In this model the clinician can list the different 'agenda' items and see where these can be easily worked out together or where conflicts need to be explored.

In this model, clinicians have the obligation to test the patient's concerns.

Knowing what the patient is concerned about

Sometimes this is easy – the patient makes his/her concerns quite clear. But sometimes it is difficult, as the patient does not lay out his/her concerns. This

---

* Acetaminophen is the American name for the same (generic) drug

might be because of embarrassment (for example, with sexual problems or some other social stigma), or simply because they cannot articulate them.

Whatever the model, patients' concerns must be elicited. How do we do this? This is not easy. This requires expertise in communication. Some can do this intuitively, others need help most of the time, and nearly everyone needs help in some situations. Structured formats of asking is one way to improve communication.[19]

The 90-seconds rule

This is to let patients talk uninterrupted (except for minimal encouragers) for the first 2 minutes of the consultation, to enable patients to feel they have expressed themselves adequately. This approach might feel to some clinicians as if it would cause unnecessary delay to the start of the consultation, but to the contrary, doing so does not increase the total length of the consultation (and most have finished their first bit of history in 90 seconds).[23]

Communication techniques

Whatever model is selected, it is useful to have some techniques perfected for helping patients to express themselves (see Table 2.4).

Good communication

How can we tell if we are communicating well? Unfortunately it is very easy to assume that all is going well. Patients are usually reluctant to say they are not happy with their doctor's performance.

Good communication = better two-way understanding; i.e., the doctor understands the patient's problem and his/her concerns, and the patient understands the doctor.

Different models of communication

There are several concepts that are important to understanding the process. Some of these ideas overlap.

Patient centred-ness

This term is used as an opposite to the traditional 'disease centred' approach. It means thinking less about the illness and more about the person suffering it. It arose out of observed consultations in which doctors seemed to have performed particularly well. What made these consultations – which struck richly important areas of concern for patients – so successful? The doctors who performed well attributed success to 'stepping into the patient's shoes'. Patient centred-ness makes it easier to understand patients' points of view: to place *their* agenda items high on the list. It also makes it easier to follow through the management part of the consultation, through with the patient's priorities

Table 2.4 Some techniques used to help patients feel enabled to talk freely about their problems.[24]

Element	Comment	Examples
Open questioning	The doctor is led to the problem by allowing the patient to control the consultation at this point in time.	'What can I do for you today?' 'Is there anything else bothering you?'
Closed questioning	The doctor retains control of the consultation so that matters high on the doctor's agenda are addressed.	'Have you ever coughed blood?' 'Before you go into that, just tell me if it is normal for you to feel sick in the morning?'
Elaboration probe	This is a technique that allows the doctor to obtain more information. It may be a question or a comment.	'How did you feel then?' 'You look sad. Is there something making you sad?' 'Some people find those symptoms very frightening.'
Minimal encourager	A general indication for the patient to continue by giving the patient 'permission' to do so.	'Mmmm' [head-nod]; (expectant facial expression, e.g., eyebrows raised).
Repeating Summarising Paraphrasing Reflecting Interpreting Confronting	(These techniques overlap, and form a continuum in which there is increasing interpretation and input from the clinician). Setting the agenda. Enabling the patient to know that the doctor has understood – and to allow the doctor to know that the patient knows this. Providing insight for the patient. Allowing the patient to address the unpalatable.	'You feel really low.' 'So the headache comes on at the back, and is worse at weekends.' '. . . and you want to make sure it couldn't be anything nasty, like cancer?' 'I've noticed that the times you've had the headache very badly seem to be when you might think your husband has been playing up.' 'You're not getting addicted to these pills, are you?' 'Do you think you will ever feel well enough to get back to work?' 'I'm worried that little Sam might be at risk from your mood swings.'

Note: These forms of communicating are not necessarily 'good' or 'bad'. They have uses in different situations. For example, open questions are good for getting started and commonly used initially in a consultation, while closed questions enable a doctor to check on important issues that the patient might not have thought to mention.

foremost. There is evidence that a patient-centred approach improves patient satisfaction, although it may not change patient health outcomes.[25]

There are instruments for measuring some elements of *patient centred-ness*.

Enablement

One problem with a patient-centred approach is the danger of accepting a patient's preferences at face value. Usually this is fine. But sometimes a clinician will help a patient by using techniques such as focussing on opportunistic prevention (especially something not presented by the patient); confronting the patient with something unpalatable; or challenging them to accept responsibility for some aspect of their illness – all things that might be unwelcome, at first, anyway.

One attempt to address this, and several other issues, is the concept of *enablement*. Here a patient goes through several steps. These include:
• Listing their health problems.
• Arranging them by priority.
• Deciding which problems need addressing at *this* consultation.
• Deciding if they had been met afterwards.
The clinician's job is to ensure the patient is enabled to get the care needed – not necessarily what they initially thought they wanted.

One problem is that in the heat of the moment with the doctor only some things get aired. Nearly half of patients have questions and issues that are not addressed in the normal course of primary care.[19] One way of dealing with this may be for clinicians always to end by asking if there's anything else – even when they already think everything is covered.

Doctor: '... And so that's good. Now, is there anything else you wanted to discuss? Nothing at all? OK then...'

Motivational interviewing

Doctors sometimes see that the best thing a patient can do to improve his or her health is to try to change the life-style. This is especially important in health promotion within the consultation (see Chapter 8 on Screening).

Those skilful in it employ all the devices talked about above, including understanding the patient's concerns and priorities, ensuring the patient's agenda is clearly foremost and yet providing enough information to alter that agenda towards what the doctor judges will provide most benefit.

Here is a worked example of a middle-aged patient who was depressed, and whose doctor realised that she would benefit by addressing a series of

Table 2.5 A series of agendas, ordered by both the doctor and the patient, with assessment of likely success (from the literature) and negotiated priority list.

Calculated medical priority list	Patient preference list	Published success rate (%)	Stage of change	Success of prior change attempts	Chance of success	Shared priority list
1 Smoking	1 Smoking	9	Contemplation	4	7	1 Depression
2 Cholesterol	2 Weight	5	Contemplation	1	4	2 Exercise
3 Exercise	3 Depression	70	Preparation	1	9	3 Smoking
4 Weight	4 Exercise	35	Contemplation	3	8	4 Alcohol
5 Alcohol	5 Alcohol	10	Precontemplation	4	6	5 Cholesterol
6 Depression	6 Cholesterol	50	Precontemplation	1	6	6 Weight

Table 2.6 Types of continuity.

System	Example	Continuity	Availability and access	Skills provided
Individual clinician	General practitioner or family physician.	√√√√	√√	√
Single practice	Team of primary care doctors, nurses and health workers.	√√√	√√√	√√√
Health maintenance organisation	Full spectrum of primary and secondary care doctors.	√	√√√	√√√√

different health threats (whose importance is assessed by some rough and ready epidemiological reckoning).[26]

It is worth noticing that the doctor's priority changed. Doctors are not 'always right'. Deciding what to do will be most successful if the patient's preferences and priorities, as well as the chances of success, are also taken into account.[26]

Continuity

This is a characteristic of care valued especially by primary care doctors. Others also believe it is important – especially in chronic illness, and psychiatric care. However, it is not quite clear what it encompasses. To some it is the traditional care provided by general practitioners and family physicians in past generations: there was one doctor you went to, who knew you, your environment and your family. The *knowing* is the important ingredient. This should include health priorities and values, which should enable better management decisions.

Continuity might mean always seeing the same individual doctor. But this means this person must be available for all care – at any time! So it has now come to mean care by a single practice of clinicians, sharing the care between them. This, in turn, has come to mean sharing one medical record, the means by which such information can be shared. It is not clear if this is effective (see Table 2.6).

Medical records and letters then become important methods of communicating between members of the unit, providing continuity.

Safety netting

This is a process for minimising problems from unexpected events or outcomes of the illness occurring after the patient has left (see Box 2.5). This was first popularised in primary care.[27] The best way to guard against such disasters is to think through the possible unexpected outcomes, and what the patient (or the patient's parents) might experience, and what they should then do.

Box 2.5 Forms of Safety-Netting

Safety net: examples	Positives	Negatives
Formal follow-up visit '...*Here's your appointment for 6 weeks*...'	Easy to establish. Can easily tell if the patient does not come	Often redundant. Irritating to patients who do not need it.
Explicit invitation '...*If your temperature is not normal by Thursday I should see you the following day*...'	Clear instructions – easy to follow	Tedious to set up
Informal blanket invitation: ' *If you have any worries, give us a call*...'	Open invitation Patients choose when a return is necessary	Patients respond too quickly or too slowly Patients concerned about deciding
Implicit invitation as part of every consultation	Automatic if there already exists a good trusting patient-doctor relationship	Most dangerous: patients may miscue when to respond

There are some extra-special forms of communication that also need to be thought of.

Medico-legal worries

One of the great concerns to doctors is the thought of being sued by a patient. This is becoming very common. It may lead to 'defensive medicine' (which usually means testing for unlikely diagnoses more often, and perhaps also offering expensive treatment – especially if of doubtful value – more often).

But there are surprises. It seems that just plain bad clinical outcomes are a rare cause of being sued. In fact, examining the clinical records among those from whom some have initiated medico-legal actions shows that it is not possible to pick those at risk. What is? It is failures in communication in about one third.[28] Another third are from offence caused by patient perceptions of arrogance or being too hurried. Unrealistic patient expectations are found in only 5%.

It is therefore important to know when the patient does not understand you, the clinician. We have already mentioned simple ways of checking this,

---

Box 2.6 Checking the Patient Understands the Clinician

- Assume nothing – always check
- Checks can be simple:
  '...Does that make sense to you...?'
- Checks can be more testing:
  '...Do you want to tell me what you understand by all that?
- Write things down:
  '...Would you like to take this diagram away with you...?'
- Arrange for a friend or relative to be there too, or suggest they tell someone about it at home
- Make opportunities for things to be checked at another visit
- Tape-record the explanation:
  '...You might want to play this to your daughter later...'

---

and it is often important to check these. Assume nothing when it comes to appreciating whether the patient has understood you (see Box 2.6).

Special communication

Bad news

One issue is disclosure. Should bad news always be told to a patient? There is still serious dispute that this is always in the patient's best interest.[29] There are some conditions when it is not best to disclose 'everything': when this might harm the patient; when they expressly do not want to know; and in emergencies (no time).[30] In several cultures it is still common practice for doctors to avoid offering shocking diagnoses (of cancer, for example).[31] Medical language has developed a complicated set of euphemisms to disguise the brutality of some diagnoses (see Box 2.7). *The Hospital of Incurable Disease* in London was renamed *Brompton Hospital* about 50 years ago.

Box 2.7 Medical Euphemisms that Disguise Some Diagnoses

Euphemism	Real meaning
'...Neoplasm...'	Cancer
'...Your baby seems to be a slow developer...'	Intellectually disabled
'...There seem to be little patches of inflammation in the spinal cord...'	Multiple sclerosis
'...Seborrhoeic keratosis...'	Senile wart
'...Hansen's disease'	Leprosy
'...Some malignant cells...'	Cancer
'...Palliative treatment...'	It is incurable
'...A bit of fluid on your lung...'	Heart failure[32]

Box 2.8 'Reframing': The Optimistic Portrayal of Dread Diagnoses

Problem	The new frame
Prostate cancer	'Most people with prostate cancer do not die of it.'
Breast cancer	'Most people with breast cancer do not die of it, and the cosmetic options are now very good...'
Genital herpes simplex, which is incurable	'...This is like a cold sore, and caused by a very closely related virus...'
HIV infection	'...This diagnosis is no longer so grim, and people can live healthily for decades now with proper treatment...'

There are, of course, two sides to this coin. Sometimes the use of euphemisms is patronising and patients feel degraded by it. But patients sometimes benefit from having the same 'truth' expressed in a more optimistic way. This is called 're-framing' (see Box 2.8).

The controversy surrounding the dispute that some established diagnoses – let alone some diagnostic possibilities – might harm some patients highlights an important point. Measuring quality only by patient satisfaction has some serious pitfalls.

When a clinician has to impart bad news, it is important to do it well. Clinicians often do it worse than policemen.[33] Some simple rules may be very helpful (see Box 2.9).

Box 2.9 How to Give Bad News

- Choose a quiet setting away from the hurly burley of the busy clinical setting
- Ensure that telephones, mobiles or bleepers cannot interrupt
- Ensure that the patient is warned and prepared:
  - '...I wonder if you could sit down...'
  - '...I am afraid I have some very bad news...'
- Make sure there is time...
  - for reflection
  - to ask questions
  - so patients do not feel hurried
  - for them to sit alone if necessary
- Attempt to find someone who can be with them afterwards

Heartsink patients
These are patients that clinicians dread. Nearly every practice that has significant continuity (primary care, and psychiatry, especially) has a few. Heartsink patients are so-called because of the sensation they engender in their carers.[34] They typically have these characteristics:
- frequent attenders;
- high consumers of health care (investigations, referrals and treatments);
- chronic conditions that are unresponsive to management.

The importance to communication is that it is important to recognise such patients because otherwise . . .
- the clinician is more prone to burn-out;
- the care delivered can be seriously sub-optimal.

The best protection is simply recognition.

> Doctor (to herself): *'Oh no: It's Angela again. I can't believe she has come round so soon! I know. I will give myself a cup of coffee afterwards, and let me just check she isn't due for her Pap smear. . . '*

CHAPTER 3

Models of disease

What we will do here is set out some models of disease, and then apply them to some clinical problems to see how the models shape up. The models of disease we discuss are not all mutually exclusive, but different ways of viewing the clinical problems we encounter. The models include:
- cause and effect models, and their several variants;
- 'edge of the distribution' illnesses (also known as 'spectrum disorders');
- spontaneously remitting and self-perpetuating illnesses; and
- 'alternative' medicine models.

These are all 'transparent box' approaches to disease: that is, a model of how the disease works, which in turn should suggest how we might treat it. But we can also take a 'black box' or empirical approach, which recognises a pattern of illness, and base treatment on what has worked with similar patterns in the past. These approaches are complementary. The models can also mislead us, and so we will also discuss the important topic of 'non-disease', that is, conditions that now or in the past have been given the label of a 'disease' but where the condition is a harmless variant of normal, or a misunderstanding of causation.

'Cause-and-effect'

Philip is a 24-year-old complaining of weight loss and thirst. He admits to getting up several times during the night to pass urine. He has an infected sore on his calf from an insect bite.

Cause-and-effect is the traditional disease model that we are most familiar with. The model suggests a specific causal agent, such as a virus, chemical or gene defect, which leads to specific disease manifestations. Such diseases have clearly defined causes with effects that can be deduced in a straightforward manner. Not every 'cause-and-effect' disease is well understood. Nor do we easily understand every mechanism. However, there is just little doubt that these illnesses *can* be explained.

Examples include infectious diseases, endocrine disorders and single gene disorders (such as PKU). Consider insulin-dependent diabetes.

Here we have an understanding of the processes: there is a failure of production of insulin for the metabolic requirement of the food intake, and blood glucose rises as predicted from an understanding of the mechanism of action of insulin. The consequences of this in the short-term are clear (polyuria and

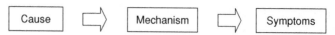

Figure 3.1 A simple cause-and-effect model.

then polydipsia) and in the long-term (glycosylated tissue being damaged and being more subject to hypoxia and necrosis). See Figure 3.1.

The examples above involve a single major cause, albeit with a chain of mechanisms leading to the outcomes and symptoms. However, often the causal process is more complicated and involves several factors, perhaps operating at different stages. For example, most cancers appear to be multifactorial with several potential initial causes (initiators), which can start the process, and with different factors speeding the process once initiated (promoters).

Melanoma probably has a mechanism like this, with several causal factors (including genetic susceptibility, number of melanocytic naevi), and the hugely important promoter, sunlight, acting to cause the damage to the cellular genetic material that results in cancer. (In this example, sunlight acts both as a causal factor – it causes an increase in melanocytes – as well as a promoter.)

Very often the mechanisms are psychological (see Figures 3.2 and 3.3). Stress may cause several psychological states, which in turn can cause physical problems too.

Notice that Table 3.1 has many question marks. There are even more question marks than indicated: why does *Meningococcus* only very rarely move from colonisation of the upper respiratory tract to the blood stream and meninges? Why does *Helicobacter pylori* infect some people and not others? Why are some people so much more susceptible to sunlight in generating melanoma than others?

As a profession we have been guilty of disguising what is not known (Table 3.2). Perhaps this is our misguided attempt at reassuring patients that their doctors know what is happening. Perhaps we are reassuring ourselves...

When patients tell us they have a sore throat, and we translate this symptom into Greek or Latin (or a mixture of both), have we really done them a service? Probably not, though some patients do find the label useful as it can smooth

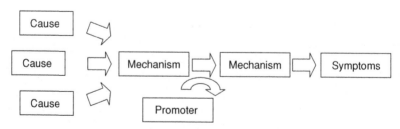

Figure 3.2 Multifactorial cause-and-effect model with several steps and a promoter.

Malfunction   Symptoms: clinical picture

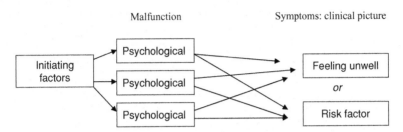

Figure 3.3 Multifactorial cause-and-effect model with several psychological steps and outcomes.

the way with relatives or their workplace; e.g., viral gastroenteritis sounds a more reasonable excuse for time off than its colloquial equivalent.

Other 'cause-and-effect' models

Cause-and-effects are not always helpful. For example people brought up under a Western medical tradition are confused by the causal models of disease offered by other cultures.

Just having a model of disease does not guarantee success at treating it. In fact to the contrary, there is renewed interest in thinking about empirical models of disease.

Table 3.1 Examples of causes and the mechanism.

Name	Symptom	Mechanism	Cause
Diabetes	Thirst, polyuria	Pancreatic failure of insulin production	?
Meningococcal meningitis	Headache, rash, photophobia, collapse	Bacterial invasion, haemorrhage	*Meningococcus*
Peptic ulcer	Epigastric pain	Decreased protection of mucosa	*Helicobacter pylori*
Tension, headache	Band-like headache	?	?
Depression	Feeling miserable, lack of energy	?	?
Melanoma of the skin	Growing black spot	Sunlight	Genetic predisposition
Irritable bowel syndrome	Abdominal pain, diarrhoea, constipation	?	?

Table 3.2 Some euphemisms for 'we don't know'.

Euphemisms	Examples
Idiopathic...	Thrombocytopaenia
Essential...	Hypertension
Primary...	Aldosteronism
Cryptogenic...	Fibrosing alveolitis
Greek name of...	Pharyngitis
Latin name of...	Tonsillitis*
Eponymous	Crohn's disease

*Etymologists should be horrified: the *tonsil-* stem is Latin, but the *-itis* suffix (meaning *inflammation)* is Greek.

Empirical disease models

Although some of the greatest advances in medical science have resulted from understanding diseases' patho-physiology (such as the role of insulin in diabetes), this is not always the case (Table 3.3). In fact medical students may be lulled into a false sense of medical science's breadth of understanding pathophysiology. More often we do not. The mechanism is not (yet) clear for many diseases.

In these cases we have to rely on simple observational information about the illness to manage it (empiricism). Many historical examples illustrate this (Table 3.4).

Indeed it was only in the twentieth century that treatments based on an understanding of mechanisms became more effective than empirical approaches. Nor even now can we rely solely on an understanding of mechanism to develop treatments. Our understanding is never complete enough, and

Table 3.3 Other 'cause-and-effect' models outside the Western tradition.

Model	Detail
The four humours: black bile, yellow bile, blood and phlegm	The earliest ancient Greek civilisation model, in which disease was an imbalance of the humours. Traces of the model still exist in our language: 'phlegmatic' (now meaning 'accepting'); sanguine (full-blooded); melancholic (sad); and choleric ('strong')
Chiropractic, osteopathy and Alexander Method	Many diseases are attributed to dysfunction of the spine or posture and its effect on the spinal nerves
Homeopathy	Based on a theory that 'like cures like', and cures are identified by giving minute doses of an agent, which in larger doses, would give the same symptoms as the disease
Spirit possession, evil humours and divine intervention	The boundaries of medicine and religion can become very blurred

Table 3.4 Some important historical empirical and effective treatments.

Disease	Empirical management	Modern interpretation
Dropsy	Foxglove extract	We now recognise this disease as heart failure, and the important ingredient as digoxin
Fever	Quinine	Quinine attacks the malaria parasite
Scurvy	Lime juice	Lind found that limes cured scurvy better than any of the several alternatives he tried, in what was probably the earliest clinical trial (see at http://www.jameslindlibrary.org/). Citrus fruit subsequently became used as a cure for over a century before the discovery of vitamin C

always requires verification with empirical testing even with good causal models. Without this we can be mislead, as with the use of Class 1 anti-arrhythmic drugs for preventing sudden death after myocardial infarction (they actually increase the sudden death rate!).

And not all treatment discoveries are based on our causal understanding – chance and observation still plays an important role. For example, the use of sildenafil for erectile dysfunction was accidentally noted while testing the use of it in patients with angina, and noting that the men were reluctant to give back any tablets.

Note: Evidence-based medicine (EBM) tests the 'cause-and-effect' model empirically.

Examples:
- Tight glycaemic control protects diabetics from small vessel disease.
- Procainamide to protect the recent myocardial infarct from arrhythmia.
- Mammography to reduce deaths from breast cancer.

Summary of the principles:
1 Understanding the mechanism of disease enables a rational approach to care.
2 Patients who understand their illness may have a better platform to help themselves.
3 Even if we (think we) understand a disease, we must still test any consequent management.

Edge-of-the-distribution illness: normal and abnormal

Jason M is a 27-year-old with anxiety. He becomes trembly when he has to stand to deliver marketing reports at work. His voice becomes dry and hoarse, and his palms are sweaty.

'I've always been a worrier,' he says. *'This is ruining my life. Why am I like it? What could have happened in my childhood to leave me like this?'*

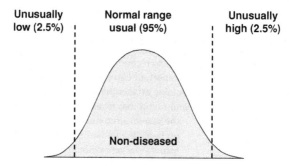

Figure 3.4 A normal distribution of a human characteristic, such as anxiety.

Anxiety and its physical symptoms are very common complaints in clinical practice. Why does it occur? The epidemiology suggests that there is rarely a clearly defined physiological or pathological cause (although sometimes rare causes such as thyrotoxicosis, phaeochromocytosis should be entertained). Anxiety is usually psychological, and some degree is a normal human feature, but with variation between people. We should think of anxiety, and similar traits, as a human characteristic that is normally distributed, as illustrated in Figure 3.4. Some people will have more, some less.

There are synonyms for 'edge of the distribution' illness, such as 'spectrum disorder'. Attention deficit hyperactivity disorder, anxiety, being tall or short etc., are all examples of spectrum disorders.

Polycythemia and anaemia are manifestations of disease caused by excess or insufficient red cells in the blood (Figure 3.5). They may cause symptoms (but not invariably). Symptoms may exist in their absence (and in the absence of any discernable abnormality of the system).

Summary of the principles:
4 Many diseases are simply extremes of the normal distribution of human characteristics.
Knowing this should help...

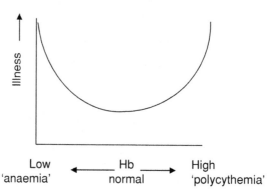

Figure 3.5 Example of the effect of the quantity of a human characteristic, in this case haemoglobin (Hb) on health.

5 . . . patients understand their problems,
6 . . . doctors do not chase futile 'causes'.
What is the dividing line between normally high and abnormally high? Why do we have 'anxiety' at all?

Anxiety is probably a characteristic selected by survival of the fittest. Our prehistoric ancestors needed some anxiety to alert them to danger. The optimal level would have been the level (not far from what is normal now) that enabled us to take the appropriate amount of caution and risk in finding food and reproducing, but without being continually frozen by fear. But this leaves room for considerable biological variation. Within this range definitions of 'normal' are arbitrary. The vertical dotted line could be set at two standard deviations (at about 2.5% above and 2.5% below) from the mean to choose a statistical version of 'normal' (Figure 3.4). But as we will see, labelling of 'dis-ease' is culturally determined. It is an arbitrary, movable line. For some people the anxiety levels are right for their environment; for others it is too high, and others again too low.

Attempts to 'explain' such diseases using the simple cause-and-effect model are littered with blind alleys. Was the whole of neurotic psycho-analysis (initiated by Freud) based on such misconceptions?

Doctor: '. . . and so Jason, it may not be helpful to look for a reason for the problem you have. There may not be a reason other than you were just born with 'too much' anxiety. Our job is to work out how we can help you overcome the symptoms. Now I have several ideas . . . '

Non-diseases

What is a disease? It is often a good idea to challenge whether a diagnostic label is a 'real' disease at all.

Sometimes a mistaken patho-physiology has caused us to create new diseases that do not exist. The best example is that of gastroptosis (see Box 3.1).

Box 3.1 Gastroptosis: An Example of a Disease That Never Existed

The name means 'dropped stomach', and was thought to be the explanation of epigastric pain in the late nineteenth century. Clinicians investigating such symptoms found people at barium swallow X-rays to have much lower stomachs than expected from autopsy examinations. An operation 'gastropexy', was devised to hitch the stomach back up to the diaphragm where it 'should' be (at autopsy!).

Other 'diseases' in the past have included homosexuality and masturbation. This points to the fact that many illnesses are culturally based. In different

Table 3.5 Some mild non-specific conditions that are culturally specific.

Malaise name	Country	Therapeutic consequences
'Off colour'	Britain	Over-use of iron replacement in the 1960s
'Mal au foie'	France	Over-use of vitamins (to support the liver)
Hypotension	Germany	Blood pressure raising drugs (such as pseudoephedrine)
'Hot' and 'cold' feelings	Vietnam	Eating compensating 'cold' or 'hot' foods to balance the ying and yang

times and cultures, diseases move in and out of the 'disease' status. Some diseases that hardly exist nowadays were once very common (such as 'swooning' of nineteenth century high class women).

Nowhere are culturally sensitive 'diseases' more apparent than in mild, non-specific manifestations of malaise (Table 3.5).

Another type of non-disease is the creation of a disorder because a treatment exists to treat it. The pharmaceutical industry has been accused of this, conducting publicity campaigns to create markets for their drugs (see Box 3.2).

Box 3.2 'Medicalisation': New 'Diseases' for Which Drugs are Available to Treat

- Male pattern baldness
- Being fat
- Menopause
- Being unhappy
- Reduced sex drive

These 'new diseases' hardly existed a generation ago. If you have trouble with this, consider the following in Box 3.3. Are they diseases?

Box 3.3 Are These Diseases?

- Being male*
- Being hung-over from alcohol
- Abstaining from alcohol completely

*Being male is associated with a lot of risk-taking and antisocial behaviour, and a very much shorter lifespan from cardiovascular disease. Some people, usually women, agree that being male *is* indeed a disease!

Table 3.6 Muddling risk factors with diseases: are these risk factors or diseases?

Hypertension	This is usually asymptomatic (symptoms are very rare nowadays, so-called 'malignant hypertension')
Diabetes	Its most important feature is the risk of complications – long-term and short-term. If associated with symptoms, it should properly be called a disease. But if not...?
Hepatitis C	Usually this does not cause symptoms. It is, however, a risk factor for liver disease decades into the future
Being male	(See Box 3.3)
Being an Australian Aborigine	This is a risk factor for much earlier death from a variety of diseases, especially cardiovascular diseases*

*Put here to emphasise the absurdity of some classifications.

Perhaps they are only risk factors. A third type of disease creation is the confusion of risk factors with disease states. Which of the conditions in Table 3.6 are diseases and which are risk factors?

Of course the notion of 'real' in disease is probably an error. 'Diseases' are short-cut words used by clinicians to summarise a constellation of symptoms and/or signs with either a specific prognosis or response to treatment. They may not be real entities. We discuss this in more detail in Chapter 4, on diagnostic reasoning.

Changes in 'normal' over the ages

Many diseases of western lifestyle derive from changes in underlying risk factors (Table 3.7).[35]

Table 3.7 Average values of physiological variables in present-day Western societies compared to probable prehistoric values (modified after Law).[35]

Physiological variable age 60	Prehistoric value	Current value	Percentage of current western population below prehistoric
BP (mmHg)			
Systolic	110	145	<1
Diastolic	70	80	<5
Serum cholesterol (mmol/l)	3.2	6.0	<1
Body mass index (BMI)	22	27	<10

These values have enormous implications when we come to think about preventing disease. See Chapter 8.

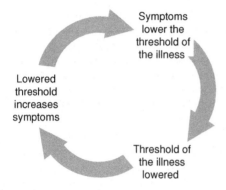

Symptoms
lower the
threshold of
the illness

Lowered
threshold
increases
symptoms

Threshold of
the illness
lowered

Figure 3.6 The positive feedback loop of self-perpetuating disease.

Self-perpetuating illness

Kim Le Tran is in an anxiety state. She is short of breath and frightened. She is complaining of pins and needles on her lips and fingertips, and she has just suffered a cramp in which her left forearm went into spasm.

If we think of spontaneously remitting diseases as being a negative feedback loop, then there is a smaller group of diseases that have a positive feedback.

These illnesses always have a subjective element to them. They exist when the threshold to the perception of 'dis-ease' is dependent on the presence of symptoms. Then the symptom-response becomes caught in a positive feedback loop (see Figure 3.6).

What does this mean? A positive feedback is a system in which the outcome of the system reinforces the process, the outcome is further increased, there is even more reinforcement so that the process escalates. Nuclear explosions are positive feedback systems.

This example is called hyperventilation. The process is well understood. Anxiety causes the person to breathe in more than their oxygen needs. Extra oxygen does not cause a problem. However, the extra loss of carbon dioxide does because this is weak acid, and the blood develops a modest rise in pH. This causes some minor disturbance of nerve function, especially the smallest diameter nerve (long sensory nerves to richly enervated areas such as lips and finger tips). The disturbance, which is caused by changes in calcium solubility – which is very pH-dependent – means that the nerves discharge more quickly,

Table 3.8 Other examples of self-perpetuating diseases.

Disease	Trigger	Self-perpetuating process
Neurodermatitis *also* pruritus ani.	Any event causing itch	Scratching causes damage, inflammation and continued itch
Chronic fatigue syndrome	Perhaps a viral infection	Creates fatigue, lack of physical activity and leads to an ongoing sense of fatigue

giving rise to the sensations of tingling lips and fingers, and even affecting the motor system (hence the tetany of the forearm).

The positive feedback loop arises because the patient finds the symptoms frightening, thereby increasing the anxiety levels. This in turn causes more over-breathing, and so the condition becomes self-perpetuating, or she collapses from exhaustion.

Understanding this model – which is really just a variant of the simple cause-and-effect model – is useful in enabling an understanding of several less simple illnesses (Table 3.8). We will enlarge on them in the treatment section.

CHAPTER 4
Diagnosis

The three main tasks of the clinician are diagnosis, prognosis and treatment. Of these, diagnosis is by far the most important for upon it the success of the other two depend.

J. A. Ryle[36]

Being able to diagnose illness is a fundamental skill in medicine. We need to know how to listen to our patients, to know which questions to ask depending on the patient's presenting problem or complaint, to determine the presence or absence of the relevant clinical signs, to know how to elicit these signs and to know which tests, if any, to order. Although diagnostic reasoning is critical to clinical practice, the way that doctors make such decisions is not well understood. Several competing theories have been proposed to describe how clinicians arrive at a diagnosis. There are also theories on how clinicians *should* use information to determine a diagnosis. This chapter looks at both what is known about diagnostic reasoning and how it might be improved. First, however, it is important to understand what clinicians are trying to do when making a diagnosis. What are we doing when we give an illness a name?

The purpose of diagnosis

When we make a diagnosis, we put the patient in a category of patients that we believe are in some way similar. For example, when we label a patient's breathing difficulty as asthma or his/her headache as migraine, the diagnostic label acts as shorthand that provides information about the likely prognosis and effects of treatment. The labels help us make management decisions. Diagnostic labels can also serve a social function, for example they allow us permission to not be at work. It is important to remember, however, that disease labels are semantic categories only. The boundaries that we place around a diagnosis or disease classification are, in fact, relatively arbitrary and disease classifications change reasonably frequently.

For example, the way that we have defined myocardial infarction has changed substantially over the past 100 years. In the first half of the twentieth century, there was a dramatic increase in the incidence of myocardial infarction in Europe and North America. Partly, this appears to be a true increase in the incidence of the disease as a result of increasing industrialisation. But it was also a result of the increasing availability of tests such as electrocardiograms, leucocyte counts and erythrocyte sedimentation rates, which

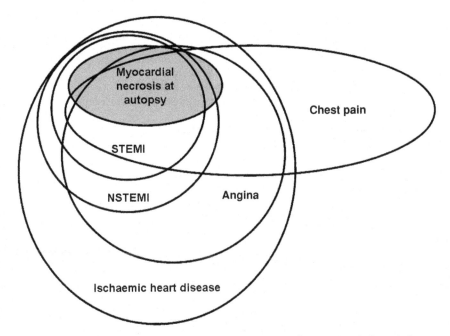

Figure 4.1 Relationship between chest pain, ECG, CK and troponins, ischaemic heart disease and myocardial infarction. (STEMI = ST elevated myocardial infarction; NSTEMI = non-ST elevated myocardial infarction.)

were able to detect the disease.[37] As we have introduced new diagnostic tests, the spectrum of patients who are diagnosed with myocardial infarction has changed (Figure 4.1). Another substantial shift has occurred in recent years with the introduction of troponin testing. There is now a new category of myocardial infarction, non-ST-elevation myocardial infarction (NSTEMI),which is troponin elevation without the traditional ECG changes of myocardial infarction. Patients with NSTEMI have a different prognosis and possibly require different treatment to patients with STEMI.

Myocardial infarction is an obvious example of diagnostic drift, but there are many others. Even diseases that seem to have a reasonably objective pathological definition, such as breast or prostate cancer, have had considerable diagnostic drift in recent years, mainly because of changes in the diagnostic tests used to detect disease. Over time our understanding of the mechanism of diseases changes, and so does our classification of disease. In 200 years' time, the current classification of disease will likely appear as quaint to the clinicians of the time as Linnaeus' genera of disease do to us now (Table 4.1). It is important to consider this diagnostic drift, because as the spectrum of patients included within a diagnostic category changes, we need to consider how this changes the prognosis and response to treatment of the new spectrum of patients.

Table 4.1 Linnaeus' classification of genera of disease.[38]

Linnaeus' genera of diseases	
Exanthematic	Feverish, with skin eruptions
Critical	Feverish, with urinary problems
Phlogistic	Feverish, with heavy pulse and topical pain
Dolorous	Painful
Mental	With alienation of judgement.
Quietal	With loss of movement
Motor	With involuntary motion
Suppressorial	With impeded motions
Evacuatorial	With evacuation of liquids
Deformities	Changed appearance of solid parts
Blemishes	External and palpable

The natural history of any disease, as originally perceived, is not necessarily the natural history of the reclassified disease.

Faergeman[37]

Diagnostic labels are useful when they help us to predict prognosis and response to treatment. They are a means of classifying patients in a way that allows us to use the inductive reasoning processes that we need to determine management, using our personal or collective experience to predict the likely natural history and the possible benefits and harms of treatment. Making a diagnosis is useful because it helps us to categorise patients in a way that can help us to make such inferences, an intermediary step for making management decisions. Sometimes we do not need the intermediary step. The presenting complaint can be sufficient to make such decisions.

An example of a clinical situation where an exact diagnostic does not help is dysuria in women. More women with dysuria will have an improvement in their symptoms if general practitioners treat all women presenting with dysuria with antibiotics, regardless of the results of urine dipstick testing.[39]

Generally, however, making a diagnosis is an important step in deciding on the correct management for a patient. Diagnosis is therefore a way of classifying or grouping together similar patients in order to make inferences about prognosis and response to treatment.

How do doctors diagnose disease?

The process of moving from the patient's presenting complaint to the diagnosis is surprisingly complicated, and remains poorly understood. Doctors appear to use several alternative processes to varying degrees, depending on clinical experience and familiarity with the problem that is presented to them. These include:

- *Pattern recognition or feature matching.* In situations that are familiar to the doctor or where all the diagnostic information is immediately available, the doctor recognises the pattern of illness in an almost sub-conscious or intuitive way.[40] The reasoning process is similar to the way that we are able to differentiate between two makes of cars, without necessarily being able to articulate all the differences in appearances between the two makes. The most obvious examples of this type of diagnosis are those that rely principally on visual clues, the 'spot diagnosis', for example the diagnosis of eczema or herpes zoster. Even quite technical information can be diagnosed in this way, for example, the interpretation of electrocardiograms.
- *Hypothetico-deductive reasoning.* When faced with a more challenging diagnostic problem, both novice and expert doctors attempt to generate a small set of possible solutions. It has been shown that doctors are only able to consider three to five possible diagnoses at one time [41] Doctors then gather information in an attempt to either confirm or exclude the hypothesised diagnoses. Each new piece of information that is gathered either increases or decreases the probability of the hypotheses under consideration. At times, the correct diagnosis is not contained within the initial list of hypotheses. As new data is gained, it may be necessary to restructure the list, although it has been shown that doctors often find it difficult to restructure from their original list of hypotheses. Within this list of hypotheses, clinicians attempt to match the presentation of the patient with their internal 'illness scripts'.[42] or 'schema'.[43]
- *Information gathering.* For many clinical presentations, the information that is initially provided is not sufficient to generate a hypothesis. For example, a patient who presents with vomiting and abdominal pain could have one of a long list of potential diagnoses. The doctor then uses a series of questions and possibly examination findings to attempt to generate a smaller and more manageable number of possible diagnoses. This information-gathering phase has often been established as a routine by the clinician for presentations of similar clinical problems. At times, the presentation of disease will be so unfamiliar to the clinician or so non-specific that no hypothesis is generated. In these cases more generic disease classifications will need to be used. Is the patient severely ill? Does the patient require referral to another clinician?

How much of each of these methods is used will depend on the clinical situation and the experience of the doctor. As they become more experienced they tend to move more towards the pattern recognition model of reasoning with routine clinical problems.

Even when faced with an unfamiliar problem, however, it is not true that taking a 'thorough' history and examination is more likely to result in an accurate diagnosis. The 'blunderbuss' method may be useful when clinical experience does not allow history taking and examination to be more directed by the presenting problem, but it is inefficient and it is difficult for junior doctors to determine the relative value of the information gathered in this way. In fact, taking a thorough history and examination can actually contribute to diagnostic errors. It has been shown that increasing the quantity, rather than the quality, of the information gathered is related to an increased rate of inaccurate diagnosis.[42] Gathering data on a few features that can discriminate who has and who does not have a disease is more likely to lead to a correct diagnosis than extensive data gathering.

Why do clinicians make diagnostic errors?

Diagnostic errors have been termed the most serious health care quality issue.[44] The Medical Defence Union in the United Kingdom reports that failure or delay in diagnosis consistently accounts for nearly one-third of notified complaints concerning general practitioners.[45] In an anonymous reporting study conducted in British hospitals, diagnostic problems accounted for 28% of reported errors, of which half were considered to be potentially very harmful.[46] These figures are likely to be underestimates, however. The diagnostic errors that are most likely to come to light are missed diagnoses where the disease has severe or fatal consequences: diseases such as meningitis, myocardial infarction, cancers or pneumonia. Many illnesses, however, will spontaneously resolve and therefore it will never be noticed if the wrong diagnosis is made. Diagnostic errors that involve falsely diagnosing a patient with a disease that they do not have can result in unnecessary treatment, but it is almost impossible to detect this type of diagnostic error. Therefore a substantial proportion of diagnostic errors will never be detected.

One study asked internal medicine specialists to retrospectively report the reasons for diagnostic errors that they were aware of over a 12-month period (see Table 4.2).

Their responses illustrate that diagnostic errors can be due to problems in clinical reasoning skills, the doctor's knowledge base, organisational difficulties

Table 4.2 Causes of diagnostic errors (in decreasing order of frequency).[47,48]

- It never crossed my mind
- I paid too much attention to *one finding*, especially laboratory results
- I didn't *listen* enough to the patient's story
- I was too much in a hurry
- I *didn't know* enough about the disease
- I let the consultant convince me
- I didn't *reassess* the situation
- The patient had *too many problems* at once
- I was influenced by a *similar case*
- I failed to convince the patient to investigate further
- I was in *denial* of an upsetting diagnosis

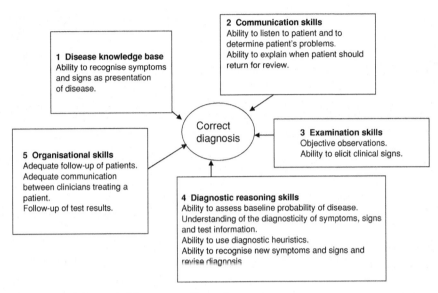

Figure 4.2 Skills needed for correct diagnosis.

or difficulties in communication between the doctor and the patient (see Figure 4.2).

The categories in Figure 4.2 may overlap. For example, a doctor may commit to the wrong diagnosis early in a clinical encounter either because of poor communication skills or because he/she has decided prematurely on a diagnosis, or both. Each of the skills in Figure 4.2 needs to be present in order for clinicians to make a correct diagnosis.

Diagnostic reasoning errors can be classified on principles of cognitive psychology: [48,49]

1 Faulty triggering
2 Faulty context formation
3 Faulty information gathering and processing
4 Faulty verification
5 'No fault' errors.

1 *Faulty triggering*: Triggering (or hypothesis generation) is the ability to develop possible diagnoses based on the presenting complaint and initial presentation of the patient. Triggering depends on the doctor's knowledge base of the symptoms associated with diseases. In a traditional sense, it is the ability to generate a list of differential diagnoses. For example, if a doctor sees a patient with palpitations, he or she needs to be able to consider the diagnosis of hyperthyroidism.

One cause for faulty triggering is that until recently, there has been a mismatch between the order in which medical information was organised and learnt and the order that it is needed in clinical practice. The traditional medical textbook is an 'encyclopaedia of disease' – divided into sections on disorders of the various organ systems with chapters on the different diseases, listing the symptoms and signs of each disease. Doctors are not, however, faced with patients with diseases, but with patients with clinical problems, often presenting in messy and atypical ways that provide misleading cues. The order in which medical information is traditionally organised is therefore not in line with the order in which it is needed to be used in clinical practice. This is slowly changing, however, with some textbooks also now presenting an 'encyclopaedia of presentations.'[49]

2 *Faulty context formation*: Context formation involves understanding the broad area and system that is the cause of the patient's symptoms. Often context errors in diagnosis involve 'premature closure', that is, the doctor begins to focus on an alternative diagnosis early in the clinical presentation and does not consider other potentially plausible diagnoses.

3 *Faulty information gathering and processing*: These errors can be subdivided into:

(a) Errors in assessment of disease prevalence. The likelihood that a clinical presentation is due to a particular disease is highly dependent on the clinical setting and the baseline probability of disease in that setting. For example, the probability that a severe headache is due to an intracranial bleed is much lower in a primary care setting than it is in an accident and emergency department. An error in judgment because of neglect of the baseline probability is termed 'representativeness bias'.[50,51]

Doctors primarily diagnose disease by matching, that is, determining how well the symptoms and signs fit with a prototypical description of the disease. This can lead to cognitive errors due to 'judging by similarity'.[52] Even if a disease presentation fits the classical picture of a rare disease, it is still more likely to be a common disease because of the baseline probability of disease. 'Rare manifestations of common diseases are more common than common manifestations of rare diseases'.[52] This is why medical students are often taught the aphorism, 'when you hear hoof-beats, think horses not zebras'.

Doctors frequently find it difficult to correctly diagnose patients when they have learnt their illness scripts in one context and then move into an unfamiliar clinical setting: for example, moving from hospital to general practice. Part of this difficulty is due to changes in the baseline probability of disease.

(b) Errors in interpretation of clinical data. Doctors can be unaware of the relative contribution of the various symptoms, signs and diagnostic test results for a diagnosis. In traditional medical textbooks, the clinical features of a disease are generally listed without mentioning which of these might be necessary or sufficient for diagnosis, let alone which symptoms or signs provide the greatest ability to rule in or rule out disease. If any information is provided, it is usually the sensitivity of a clinical finding, that is, the frequency of the finding in the diseased population. Specificity, which is the frequency of a clinical finding in a non-diseased population and which is also necessary for diagnostic decision making, is rarely given.

Much of doctors' understanding regarding the ability of clinical information to rule in or rule out disease is gathered as a result of clinical experience. However, experience may not be an accurate teacher.

'If our case numbers were truly vast (hundreds, if not thousands), if the spectrum of disease we had seen was sufficiently wide and representative, if we had used diagnostic criteria consistently over time, if we had searched for each clinical finding equally diligently in every patient, and if our memories were perfect, then perhaps our library of remembered cases would allow us to accurately estimate the frequencies of clinical manifestations of that disease and interpret them properly.'[53]

Studies of medical students and junior doctors have shown that the most common error in diagnostic reasoning is the use of non-discriminatory findings to support a diagnosis, that is, there is an error in their knowledge base which causes them to focus on a sign or symptom that is not able to accurately validate a diagnosis.[54–56] Unfortunately, this is not just a problem of inexperience. From studies examining the cognitive processes used in diagnostic decision making, physicians have difficulties in recognising the ability of information to contribute to a diagnosis and fail to select normatively optimal information.[55] This means that the clinical data that doctors collect from their history taking and examination may not be 'optimal' in terms of its ability to determine if a patient does or does not have a disease.

Doctors often place too much emphasis on a particular finding from the history, examination or investigation results, especially the ability of a test result to rule in or rule out disease.[55,57] A common error is to believe that a positive test result for an uncommon or rare disease indicates that a patient truly has the disease, even though given the baseline probability of disease it is more likely to be a false positive test result.

Doctors tend to use confirming strategies rather than disconfirming strategies and fail to understand the importance of negative information, resulting in a confirmation bias.[58,59]

Doctors anchor their probability of a specific disease early in the diagnostic process and do not revise their estimates of the probability of a diagnosis in the light of new information by as much as would be implied by probability theory. This 'conservatism' results in biases in the process of diagnosis.[60] Doctors also give more weight to information that is presented earlier in the consultation.[61,62]

(c) Errors in applications of clinical axioms. Another source of error can be the use of heuristics. A heuristic is a rule of thumb that allows a decision maker to decide on one course of action or another without needing to consider all the possible information that could be gathered and used to make that decision. To illustrate, suppose we are presented with a small yellow bird and need

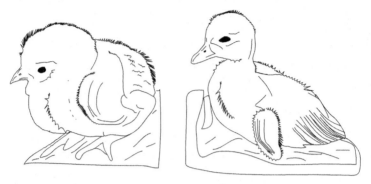

Figure 4.3 How did we make the diagnosis of these two young birds?

to decide if it is a chicken or a duck. Based on past experience or research evidence, or both, we may know that small yellow birds with webbed feet are ducks and with four-toed feet are chickens. In deciding whether this is a chicken or a duck, we may therefore not look at every possible feature that can differentiate a chicken from a duck, but may look at the bird's feet and on the basis of this make our decision (see Figure 4.3).

Experienced doctors commonly use heuristics in their diagnostic thinking.[63] For example, when a patient presents with back pain, doctors will look specifically for symptoms that may indicate a malignancy, such as pain at night. If such features are not present, the doctor will move on to other possible causes of back pain. Heuristics are extremely useful and make diagnosis a less time-consuming exercise, but being rules of thumb, they carry the risk of not always leading to the right conclusion. Few symptoms, signs and test results completely discriminate between diagnostic categories. To begin with, because of the extraordinary variety of ways in which illness can present, doctors are constantly faced with the possibility of a four-toed duck. In real life, there is no such thing as a 'typical' patient. There will be elements of the disease missing and extra features thrown in 'just to make it difficult.' Doctors therefore need to be aware of the potential errors in the use of such heuristics.

> *When I tried to teach the art of medical diagnosis to students, I often used to ask them this riddle from my prep school days: 'What runs about farm yards, flaps its wings, lays eggs and barks like a dog? It is difficult isn't it? Have you guessed it? The answer is "a hen!" Usually one of the more earnest and innocent of the students would say: 'But sir! I don't understand the bit about barking like a dog.' 'Ah yes. I must explain. That was just put in to make it difficult.'*

Asher[64]

4 *Faulty verification*: Verification involves ensuring that all the symptoms experienced by the patient are explained by the final diagnosis and that no other reasonable diagnostic possibility still exists. Verification is particularly important in situations where the disease presentation changes over time.

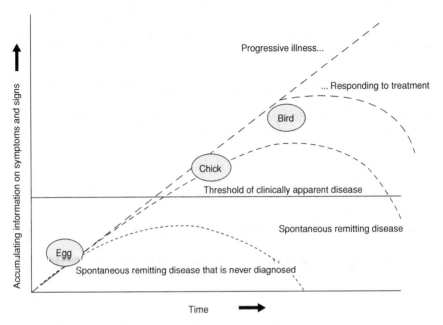

Figure 4.4 The clinical presentation of a disease over time.

Features of the illness may not be present in the early stages and the frequency and pattern of symptoms over time can be important features that help us to determine or revise our diagnosis (see Figure 4.4).

Patients often present to general practitioners at an early stage in their illness, when it can be impossible to make a diagnosis with certainty. In the early stage of an illness, there may be a large number of plausible diagnoses. Specialists may see chickens and ducks, general practitioners usually see eggs. Testing for rarer diseases at an early stage of an illness will often be inappropriate. Such a strategy is not only costly, but it also places the patient at the risk of harms both directly from the test (or any further testing that might be required) and the risk of false positive and false negative test results. When the probability of the disease is low, a positive test result at this stage is more likely to be a false positive than indicate that the patient truly has a disease. Over time, the pattern of the illness may change and the probability of a particular disease may increase. An important part of the consultation that can easily be forgotten is to communicate with patients about the expected course of an illness, and what features should cause them to present for review.

5 No-fault errors in diagnosis: Finally, the clinical presentation may be so atypical or the disease in question so rare that it is unlikely that any doctor would think of it as a diagnosis: the 'no-fault error'.[50] In the early stages of an illness, the presenting features may be non-specific and it is therefore also a 'no-fault error' to diagnose the most common form of illness with these presenting features at that stage, which only later declares itself to be a rarer cause. This type of diagnostic error cannot be prevented by improving clinical reasoning or evidence.

Differences between experts and novices

Expert clinicians collect less data when faced with a clinical problem, but are more discriminating in the information that they collect. They are able to generate accurate diagnostic hypotheses earlier in the clinical interview than do junior doctors, and are more skilled in gathering the information necessary for the clinical problem.[65]

Non-experts tend to use the information gathering approach when trying to make a diagnosis, rather than pattern recognition or strategies to confirm a hypothesis.[48] This approach is helpful when facing a problem that is not familiar, but it is less successful for generating specific hypotheses. Junior doctors have been found to place greater reliance on matching cases based on similarity, rather than basing their diagnosis on the ability of the features that are present and absent to rule in or rule out disease.[66]

Intuition and diagnosis

In his book on naturalistic decision making, Klein describes how 'intuition' saved the lives of a fire crew:[6]

> *'It is a simple house fire in a one-storey house in a residential neighbourhood. The fire is in the back, in the kitchen area. The lieutenant leads his hose crew into the building, to the back, to spray water on the fire, but the fire just roars back at them.*
>
> *"Odd," he thinks. The water should have more of an impact. They try dousing it again, and get the same results. They retreat a few steps to regroup. Then the lieutenant starts to feel as if something is not right. He doesn't have any clues; he just doesn't feel right about being in that house, so he orders his men out of the building – a perfectly standard building with nothing out of the ordinary.*
>
> *As soon as his men leave the building, the floor where they have been standing collapses. Had they still been inside, they would have plunged into the fire below.'*

When asked why he had made the decision to evacuate, the fire commander did not know that the house had a basement or that this was the seat of the fire, but he was able to identify that the fire did not react as he expected when sprayed with water, and that the lounge room was much hotter than he would have expected for a fire in a single-family home and that the fire was unusually quiet. The whole situation 'did not seem right'.

I had a similar experience one Saturday morning when filling in for a doctor who was away on holidays. Half way through the morning, the practice receptionist came in and told me that a mother had brought in her 17-year-old son. He was feeling quite unwell and had asked to lie down, so she had placed the boy and his mother in the treatment room until I could see them. This immediately struck me as odd: teenage boys do not come to the general practitioner often and when they do they generally seem to minimise their symptoms. I saw the boy as the next patient. He had had symptoms of a flu-like illness for the previous 3 days and was now feeling short of breath. Given this history, the most likely diagnosis is asthma, or more uncommonly pneumonia. When I listened to his chest, however, the breath sounds were normal. Now I was worried – the situation 'did not seem right'. My knowledge base was not good enough, however, to know what might be the cause of this boy's symptoms. I thought about getting a chest X-ray at the local radiologist, but I was worried that I might not get the result until Monday. I decided to send the boy and his mother to the local children's hospital, despite the long wait that this might involve. At the end of my session I rang the hospital to ask how the boy was. The paediatric registrar came to the phone and asked me several times what was it that had made me send the boy to the hospital. I now began to feel unsure why I had sent the boy and thought maybe I had missed something obvious. As it turned out, however, the chest X-ray had shown a mediastinal lymphoma. The registrar was curious what it was in the boy's history and examination that had made me think that something was not right.

This story could have easily gone another way. Also, if I had known that patients with mediastinal lymphomas classically present with flu-like symptoms and shortness of breath, I would have referred the patient for investigation routinely and my intuitive guess would have been much less memorable for me. And of course, I have chosen to remember and write about a story where my intuition resulted in the correct diagnosis, not the times when my intuition has failed or where I have continued to treat a patient believing they have one diagnosis when it should have become clear that this was not the case.

Methods to improve diagnostic reasoning: heuristics, probabilistic reasoning and increased feedback on the reasoning process

Three methods have been proposed to improve the ability of doctors to efficiently and effectively gather diagnostic information: the use of heuristics (including Murtagh's red flag system), increased use of probabilistic reasoning and increasing the feedback to junior doctors and medical students on their diagnostic reasoning.

Heuristics and Murtagh's red flag system

As explained above, heuristics are short-cuts or rules of thumb. Experienced doctors commonly use these approaches when making a diagnosis. Junior doctors are often aware that more experienced doctors are using these short-cuts but are not often explicitly taught these methods, and importantly their limitations.

One example of a heuristic is Murtagh's red flag system.[34,67,68] This Australian general practitioner developed a method for ensuring that severe diseases are not missed in his practice. One of the great skills in primary care settings is being able to detect the severe or life threatening illness from the much more common disorders that primary care doctors see most of the time. For each clinical presentation, Murtagh listed a small number of possible diagnoses that are 'serious and not to be missed.' Doctors screen for these disorders by asking specifically about red flag symptoms or searching for red flag signs. These symptoms and signs have a high sensitivity. If they are absent, it is possible to exclude the disorder with reasonable confidence. For example, if a patient presents with back pain, it is important to exclude a neoplastic or infectious cause for the pain. The doctor can do this by asking about symptoms such as pain at night, night sweats and a past history of cancer.

This method is extremely useful for ensuring that severe diseases are not missed. The main limitation of the method is that as yet there is not a good evidence-base for determining what are the most appropriate red flag symptoms and signs for many conditions. Some important diseases do not appear to have any red flag symptoms or signs

Another useful heuristic is understanding the time course of different types of illnesses. For example, vascular events present very quickly, infection, inflammation or metabolic illness presents over hours to days and neoplastic diseases over weeks to months.[69] Understanding the typical time course of illnesses can assist in determining the type of disease that a patient has.

Probabilistic reasoning

Doctors make decisions whether patients should be started on treatment using their qualitative assessments of a patient's probability of disease. We can never be absolutely certain that a patient has a disease (whether this is recognised or not), but we are certain enough that a patient has a disease that we believe it will benefit the patient to commence treatment. One method for overcoming some of the diagnostic errors described above could be a greater use of quantitative estimates that can more accurately estimate a patient's probability of disease.

The theory of probabilistic reasoning is based on Bayes' theorem. Reverend Bayes was an eighteenth-century English cleric who developed a mathematical formula for calculating how to revise the probability of an event in the light of new information (see Figure 4.5). In the case of diagnosis, we begin with some assessment of the probability a patient has a disease based on the prevalence of disease in the local area and other more subjective factors. As we accumulate further clinical information, such as the results of diagnostic tests, Bayes' theorem allows us to calculate the revised probability of disease.

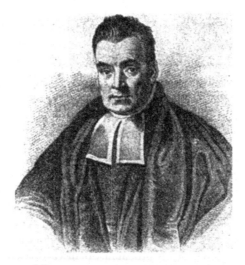

Figure 4.5 The Reverend Bayes.

The basic form of the theorem is a series of conditional probabilities. For example, the probability of a disease given a positive test result is:

$$P\left(D^{+}\,|\,T^{+}\right) = \frac{\left[P\left(T^{+}\,|\,D^{+}\right) \times P\left(D^{+}\right)\right]}{\left[P\left(T^{+}\,|\,D^{+}\right) \times P\left(D^{+}\right)\right] + \left[P\left(T^{+}\,|\,D^{-}\right) \times P\left(D^{-}\right)\right]}$$

where

$P\left(D^{+}\right)$ = prior probability of disease

$P\left(D^{-}\right)$ = probability of non-disease

$P\left(D^{+}\,|\,T^{+}\right)$ = post-test probability of disease, D^{+}, given a positive test result, T^{+}

$P\left(T^{+}\,|\,D^{+}\right)$ = probability of a positive test result, T^{+}, given the disease is present D^{+}

$P\left(T^{+}\,|\,D^{-}\right)$ = probability of a positive test result, T^{+}, given the disease is absent D^{-}

In epidemiological terms, $P\left(T^{+}\,|\,D^{+}\right)$ is the sensitivity and $P\left(T^{-}\,|\,D^{-}\right)$ to the specificity of the test. The above equation is therefore equivalent to:

Post-test probability given a positive test result =

$$\frac{(\text{sensitivity} \times \text{prior probability})}{(\text{sensitivity} \times \text{prior probability}) \times [(1 - \text{specificity}) \times (1 - \text{prior probability})]}$$

This is also equivalent to:

$$\frac{\text{true positives}}{(\text{true positives} + \text{false positives})}$$

or the positive predictive value of the test.

To use Bayes' theorem, therefore, requires knowledge of the baseline probability of disease and the sensitivity and specificity of diagnostic tests. Often clinicians do not know the exact probabilities, but develop an intuitive understanding of the probability of diseases from their experience in their own clinical setting. Even so, these intuitive assessments can be improved by more reliable data. For example, what would you say is the probability that a woman aged 60 who presents with a breast lump to her doctor has breast cancer?

The starting point for estimating the baseline probability of disease may come from published reports of the prevalence of the disease. The prevalence of a disease in a population, however, is an estimate of how likely a randomly selected person would have the disease, not the likelihood that a person who presents with a clinical problem has the disease. The probability that over a 12-month period women aged between 50 and 64 develop breast cancer is approximately 0.6%.[70] The fact that our patient presents to the general practitioner with a breast lump raises the probability of the disease to 17%.[71] We might also adjust our baseline probability of disease based on other factors. How would you assess her probability of disease if she is taking hormone replacement therapy? Or if she has a sister who has been diagnosed with breast cancer?

Diagnostic mammography has a sensitivity of 90% and a specificity of 73%.[72] Given this information, what do you think the probability of a breast cancer is if this woman has a positive mammogram?

There are several ways to calculate this, but one of the easiest is to construct a 2 × 2 table using a hypothetical cohort of 1000 patients (see Table 4.3):

If the woman has a positive mammogram, the probability that she has breast cancer is estimated by the number of true positive test results divided by all positive results, i.e., 153/377 = 40%. From this we can calculate that the given a pre-test probability of disease of 17% and a sensitivity of 90% and a

Table 4.3 The probability of breast cancer in women presenting with a breast lump.

	Disease	No disease	Total
Mammogram +ve	(Total disease × sensitivity) TP 153	(Total disease × (1 − specificity)) FP 224	Positive results 377
Mammogram −ve	(Total disease × (1 − sensitivity)) FN 17	(Total disease × specificity) TN 606	Negative results 623
	1000 × pre-test probability 170	1000 × (1 − pre-test probability) 830	1000

TP = true positive, FP = false positive, FN = false negative, TN = true negative

specificity of 73% for diagnostic mammography, the post-test probability of disease after a positive mammogram is 40%.

It is also important to consider that the post-test probability of disease if the woman has a negative mammogram. This is equal to the number of false negative results divided by all negative results. This is 17/623, which is 3%, a level that is too high for reassurance that she does not have breast cancer.

Whether the test is positive or negative, we are not able to feel that we have ruled in or ruled out the disease sufficiently, and we would go on to perform a fine needle aspiration. In some situations, however, we do not have another confirmatory test available, and we may have to accept treatment decisions with less certainty about the diagnosis.

We discuss this further in relation to Screening in Chapter 8.

Methods for incorporating probabilistic reasoning into clinical practice

As seen from the formula above, it is difficult to convert pre-test probabilities to post-test probabilities without doing some quite tedious calculations. A mnemonic helps clinicians remember when a test is useful for ruling in or ruling out disease.[72] As a generalisation, if a test has a high sensitivity and the test result is negative, it rules out disease (SnNOut). If a test has a high specificity and the test result is positive, it rules in disease (SpPIn). Note that these are generalisations. When the pre-test probability is low, even if a test has a high specificity, the post-test probability of a disease after a positive result can still be quite low. In this case, the test is not sufficiently sensitive or specific to rule in or rule out the diagnosis.

Likelihood ratios may be easier to use intuitively. The positive likelihood ratio of a test is the probability of a positive test result in the diseased population divided by the probability of a positive test result in the non-diseased population (and is equal to (sensitivity/1 – specificity). As a guide, if the positive likelihood ratio is greater than 2, it is helpful for ruling in disease and if it is greater than 10, it is very good for ruling in a disease. The negative likelihood ratio is the probability of a negative test result in the disease population divided by the probability of a negative test result in the non-diseased population (1 – sensitivity/specificity). If the negative likelihood ratio is less than 0.5, it is helpful for ruling out disease and if it is less than 0.1, it is very good for ruling out disease. Diagnostic mammogram has a positive likelihood ratio of 3.3 and a negative likelihood ratio of 0.14. It is therefore only moderately good at ruling in or ruling out disease.

Another way to quickly calculate post-test probabilities is by using a probability revision graph. These graphs convert pre-test probability to the post-test probability using the likelihood ratios of the test (Figure 4.6).

These graphs also can show the effect of combining diagnostic tests. For example, we can show the probability of disease using the possible combinations of mammography and fine needle aspiration cytology results (see Figure 4.7).

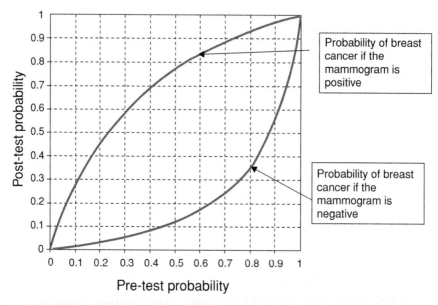

Figure 4.6 Pre-test and post-test probability curves. (See Chapter 8 on Screening).

Using the pre-test–post-test graph, we can see that there is a high probability of breast cancer if both the mammogram and biopsy results are positive, intermediate probabilities if one test is positive and the other is negative and almost zero probability of disease if both tests are negative.

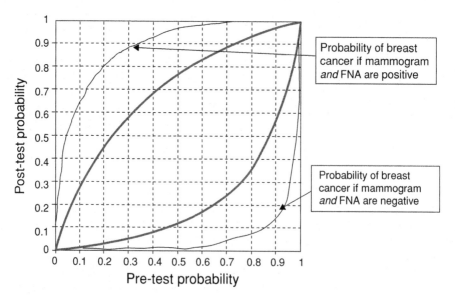

Figure 4.7 Pre-test and post-test graph of combined mammography and fine needle aspiration biopsy results for breast cancer (FNA = fine needle aspiration cytology).

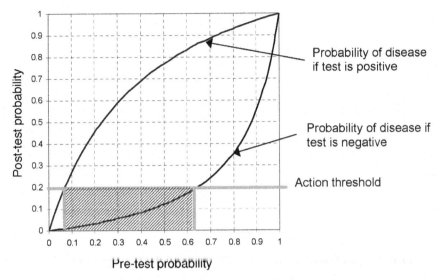

Figure 4.8 Determining the no test-test-treat thresholds for a diagnostic test.

Test ordering decisions

Diagnostic tests are of most value when the test result could lead to a change in the management of a patient. Probabilistic reasoning can help us decide when it is of value to order a diagnostic test.

The management of a patient depends on the consequences of treating or not treating the disease. There will be potential harms and benefits of treating the patient if they do have a disease (compared with not treating) and the potential harms and benefits of treating the patient if they do not have a disease (compared with not treating). We can use these probabilities to determine the action threshold, which is the probability of disease at which it becomes worthwhile to treat. For many diseases, the potential harms of treating an illness even if the diagnosis is not present is much greater than the potential harm of not treating an illness that is present. The action threshold is therefore quite low for many diseases. For example, we should treat any patient with suspected meningitis even when the probability of disease is very low, probably less than 1%.

Once we have set the threshold level at which it becomes worthwhile to treat a disease, we can determine whether we should order a diagnostic test based on the pre-test probability of the disease and the diagnostic accuracy of the test. We will illustrate how we can determine this by using a hypothetical example (see Figure 4.8).

In this case, it is worthwhile to treat the disease if the probability of disease is greater than 20%. If the pre-test probability of disease is greater than approximately 65%, we would treat the patient even if the result of the test is negative. If the pre-test probability of disease is less than approximately 7%, we would not treat the patient even if the test is positive. It is therefore only useful to use this test in the gray zone between these two values. The test will be of most value when the pre-test probability is around the value of the action threshold (that is at about 20%).

This approach can explain why diagnostic tests can be useful for investigating a symptom in one clinical setting and not in another. CT and MRI scans can detect intra-cranial causes of headaches, such as intra-cranial bleeding or tumours. In primary care settings, the pre-test probability of these diseases is very low. Therefore it would only be in cases where there were highly unusual features of the headache that it would be appropriate to investigate a patient with headache with a CT or MRI scan in this setting. The pre-test probability of intra-cranial disease is much higher in an emergency room setting. Therefore it would be appropriate to use this test in a much higher proportion of patients, possibly even all patients presenting with headache to an emergency department.

Would using Bayesian probability revision improve diagnosis and the ordering of diagnostic tests?

Doctors do revise their estimates of the probability of disease based on new information, but it has been shown that doctors consistently make errors in this process. In particular, doctors over-estimate the information that is gained from laboratory and imaging results. This can result in misdiagnosis because of the unfounded faith in test results, and causes the over-use of tests, resulting in increasing health care costs and potential harm to patients. The ordering of tests 'just to be certain' has led to a new medical syndrome, VOMIT (victims of modern imaging technology).[73]

Because of the cognitive errors in diagnostic reasoning and our over-reliance on diagnostic test results, it may be that incorporating greater use of probabilistic revision will allow more accurate estimates of the probability of disease and more rational ordering of diagnostic tests. It should be stressed, however, that we do not have a way of doing this at present. It is also important to remember that much of the information that we learn to process as doctors is in the form of what is called 'soft' data, including the non-verbal clues that clinicians can detect: does this child look sick, is it reasonable for a child with this disease to be quiet while we examine them and so forth. It is important to not forget the importance of this sort of information in our clinical reasoning.

Both doctors and patients need to accept that a certain degree of uncertainty will always be present in medical diagnosis. No approach – including the 'test for everything' approach – will be right all the time. Even as we attempt to decrease our uncertainty by ordering more tests, we incur the risk of a false positive test result and the possible consequences of treating a disease that the patient either did not have or would never have known that they had. Searching for certainty is not in the best interest of the patients or society. Doctors need the skills to assess when it is worthwhile to order a test and when it is important to stop looking, and how to communicate these decisions to their patients. We need to focus more on the patient's problems and less on coming up with the right diagnosis. Rather than attempting a fruitless quest for certainty, doctors need to be able to make decisions in the context of diagnostic uncertainty and be prepared to continually re-evaluate their decisions.

Teaching of diagnostic reasoning

In most medical schools, there is very little explicit teaching of diagnostic reasoning.[74] Students and junior doctors gain experience and skills in diagnostic reasoning primarily by observation of more senior doctors while on clinical placements.

There is some evidence that the most effective way for students to gain diagnostic skills is by practice on actual or hypothetical cases, while receiving feedback on their performance.[6,75] Essential features appear to be both the practical experience (the gaining of the stories and prototypes) and the feedback (so that abstract models and generalisations can be acquired). Students need to be exposed to a wide variety of common presentations and spectra of disease, so that they can acquire the 'illness scripts' necessary to be able to come to a diagnosis.[76] Using simulated cases with the explicit explanation of hypothesis testing and refinement and gradual release of findings, allowing students to practice their clinical reasoning appears effective.[59]

Students need to gain feedback in a wide variety of clinical contexts. This context needs to be as similar as possible to the context in which the student will work, as there is evidence that it is difficult to transfer clinical reasoning from one context to another.[77]

There should also be a movement away from the emphasis on medical students taking a 'thorough history and examination' towards the strategies that experienced clinicians actually use. At the same time, we need to ensure that students and junior doctors do not focus on a possible diagnosis too early. With the increasing availability of more tests and more expensive tests, we need to encourage students to learn not only the facts of medicine, but also the diagnostic reasoning that is necessary to practice as a safe and effective doctor.

CHAPTER 5

Fine art of prognostication

The art of the physician consists of entertaining the patient until nature cures him or her.

Voltaire

Among patients' expectations is that the doctor will be able to give them an appropriate label: 'You have X disease.' Why is this label important to both patients and doctors? For doctors, the diagnostic label is a keyword to access information – either memorised or from external sources – about the management of the condition. For the patient, the first important thing is the meaning of the label, which is the natural history of the condition. Imagine a patient's relief when you are able to say of a skin lesion, 'It's not cancer; it's just a benign lump.' The relief is linked to the prognosis. Much work in general practice is based on helping patients to understand the most likely course of their disease, even when treatment is not necessary or not possible. Consider the following four cases (see Box 5.1).

In each of these examples, an important step in management is to understand the natural history of the disease and to be able to communicate this to the patient. A good question to ask is 'What would happen if we did nothing?' The answer to this question is the natural history.

A clinician therefore needs an understanding of the nature and types of prognosis; a knowledge of the prognosis of individual conditions; and skills in expressing and communicating this to patients.

A simple communication process to explain natural history and integrate it with decision about treatment can be guided by the following three steps:

- *What would happen if we did nothing?*
  We may begin explaining the disease by saying something like: '*Do you know about X? OK, well let me explain. If we did nothing the usual course of the illness is to . . .*'
- *Explain what the options are:*
  We next list and explain the main management options, for example: 'There are three common things we can do about this: a pill, or surgery, or we can let it take its course (natural history)'.
- *Check the patient's expectations and ideas:*
  We should know if the patient has tried any of the options, or has prior knowledge and expectations about them. For example, '*Have you tried anything yourself, or did you have a preference for one of those options?*' At this

---

Box 5.1 Some illustrative cases

1 A middle-aged man is diagnosed with mesothelioma of the lung, and wants to know how long he might be expected to live.

2 A young girl with a scaly rash. It started about a week ago, and has spread alarmingly across her body.

3 A 50-year-old man has recently passed a ureteric calculus (kidney stone), and is worried about the chance of it happening again.

4 A middle-aged woman presents with pain on movement of her elbow which you diagnose as lateral epicondylitis ('Tennis elbow').

---

point a dialogue may ensue about the pros and cons of the various options, or the patient may simply ask what you recommend.

These steps correspond to the steps you learnt about earlier for decision making generally: the Problem (PRO), Alternative Actions (ACT), and Integrate Evidence and Values (IVE). We will consider later in this chapter how we should consider the management options for different patterns of disease prognosis, but first we need to think about how we predict prognosis.

Prognostic uncertainty

Using and giving a prognosis would be relatively simple if disease always followed a fixed time-scale. It does not. Prognosis, like life generally, is usually complicated by uncertainty. We may know an average, but few people are 'average,' so we need means to cope with and communicate the variations. Consider Stephen Jay Gould's story, 'The Median is not the Message'.

'In July 1982, I learned that I was suffering from abdominal mesothelioma, a rare and serious cancer usually associated with exposure to asbestos. When I revived after surgery, I asked my first question of my doctor and chemotherapist: "What is the best technical literature about mesothelioma?" She replied, with a touch of diplomacy (the only departure she has ever made from direct frankness) that the medical literature contained nothing really worth reading.'

So Gould was probably asking several questions including our first two steps above: the natural history and the further treatment options (this is a bit confusing as he describes having surgery above – was it exploratory?) Unfortunately, he did not get that information from his doctor, but instead went to the medical library at Harvard where he worked. What he found was not good news.

'An hour later, surrounded by the latest literature on abdominal mesothelioma, I realized with a gulp why my doctor had offered that humane advice. The literature couldn't have been more brutally clear: mesothelioma is incurable, with a median mortality of only eight months after discovery.'

At first sight he took this like we might a pronouncement from a mythical TV doctor who says, 'You have 8 months to live.' But it soon dawned on him that the 8 months was a point in an ocean of uncertainty.

'What does median mortality of eight months signify in our vernacular? I suspect that most people, without training in statistics, would read such a statement as, 'I will probably be dead in eight months' – the very conclusion that must be avoided, since it isn't so, and since attitude matters so much.'

A median of 8 months merely means that half those with the diagnosis will live less than that time, but (very importantly) half will live more. And the shape of that 'more' can be important too. Gould finally noted that:

'I immediately recognized that the distribution of variation about the eight-month median would almost surely be what statisticians call "right skewed".'

So that 'some' who survive that first 8 months may live substantially longer. In Gould's case it was 20 years after the diagnosis! And even then he died of another condition unrelated to his original mesothelioma. So learning to give a prognosis that also captures our uncertainty is important to manage expectations and hope.

How to express prognosis/risk

To develop an understanding of the probabilistic nature of a natural history let us begin with the natural history of people without current disease. We all have a 'prognosis', depending on our age, gender, current or past illness and a variety of personal and environmental risk factors. Actuaries put this information into life tables. It is worth understanding how to read these, as the issues are similar for the well and the diseased.

Normal life expectancy

First we need to look at life expectancy curves (see Figure 5.1).

From this you can read off several useful pieces of information. For example, the median survival is the 50th percentile, i.e., half of us live longer and half of us live less then this time point. For males it is about 78 years and for females it is 83 years. But of course, this is just an 'average': some people die as neonates and some people live to over 100. So we might say a newborn male has 78 years to live, but realise there is a considerable range to that figure!

How would you summarise these curves in Figure 5.1? We will answer the following questions from the data given in the Figure:

1 What is the median (50%) survival for (a) males and (b) females?
2 Why is the *median* survival different to the *mean* survival (the life expectancy)?

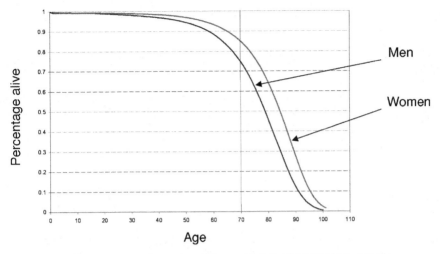

Figure 5.1 Life expectancy curves for males and females (UK life table 2002).

3 What is the absolute risk difference in mortality between men and women at age 70 years?

4 What is the relative risk of death for being male versus female at age 70 years?

The *median* survival is the 'halfway' point, at which half the population are dead and half are still alive. So we can read this off by following along from the 0.5 point on the vertical axis to each of the male and female lines, and then follow these down to the age axis to work out that males have a median life expectancy of 80 years whereas females have one closer to 85 years. Both of these values are higher than the mean or average 'life expectancy' because our natural history is 'left skewed' – the reverse of Gould's position. That is, as we age, our chances of surviving each year get less rather than more.

The absolute difference between men and women's mortality at 70 years is about 0.1 (see the solid line marked in the Figure) or 10%. The relative risk depends on whether we take a mortality or survival ratio. The mortality ratio is about $0.15/0.25 = 0.60$, that is, women only have 60% of the mortality of men by the age of 70 years (but do not think that having a gender change will reverse this, guys!).

The shape of these life expectancy curves has changed over the centuries. With improvements in infant mortality and the control of many infectious diseases, the curves have 'rectangularised', that is, the early mortality has diminished greatly, but the late mortality has diminished less (Figure 5.2). Hence most of our change in life expectancy has come from not dying early, rather than longer post-retirement years.

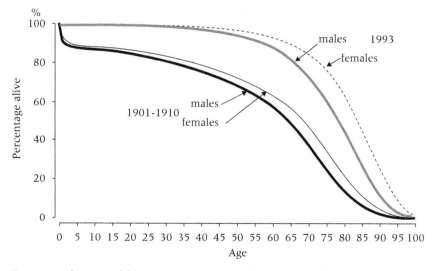

Figure 5.2 Changes in life expectancy over time. Source: Australian Bureau of Statistics. Australian Social Trends 1995.

One point to note about these life expectancy curves is that the mortality rate increases with time. That is, we have an 'accelerating' mortality. This acceleration is not perfectly constant, but, as an approximation . . .

> Mortality doubles about every 6 years

This gives us a useful alternative for expressing relative risks. If someone's relative risk of death has doubled (for example, smokers, who have a slightly greater than doubled relative risk for many conditions) then they have the mortality rate of someone 6 years older than their calendar age.

Patterns of prognosis

As we indicated at the start of this chapter, a question most patients will want answered for a new diagnosis is: *What will happen if I do nothing?* This is the natural history of the condition: the changes that will occur over time if no treatment is given. For a cold this might be a 7-day illness; for a basal cell cancer, a steady slow growth in size; and for hypertension a small but important risk of cardiovascular events such as stroke or myocardial infarction.

We can classify diseases based on the pattern of the prognosis: for example, spontaneously remitting, progressive, recurrent or intermittent and chronic (see Table 5.1 and Figure 5.3).

Although these are convenient mental boxes, remember the boundaries between them are not always clear: some diseases sit astride the boundaries. For example, psoriasis can be intermittent (clearing fully at times) or chronic and fluctuating. Tennis elbow usually clears spontaneously, but sometimes

Table 5.1 Examples of different prognoses.

Type of natural history	Examples
Spontaneously remitting	Cold, sprain, tennis elbow, gastroenteritis
Recurrent/intermittent	Migraine, vaginitis, asthma, vertigo
Chronic or fluctuating	Eczema, ulcerative colitis, rheumatoid arthritis, anxiety, hernia, irritable bowel syndrome
Progressive	Osteoarthritis, COPD, most cancers, primary biliary cirrhosis, Alzheimer's disease, Parkinson's disease, glaucoma

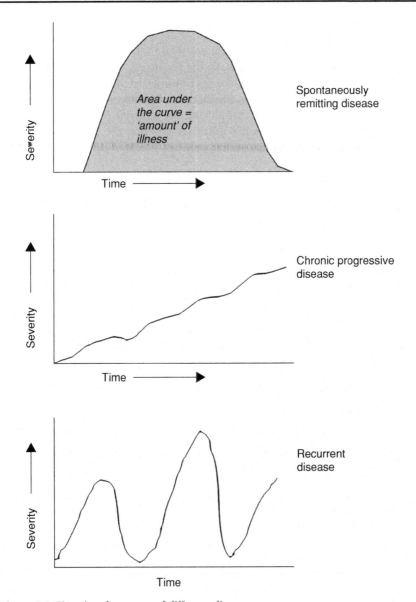

Figure 5.3 Picturing the course of different diseases.

can take months or years and may recur. Many chronic diseases are slowly progressive over time.

However, the general classification is useful. When we consider the management of a condition (as in the next chapter), and weigh up the potential benefits and harms of various treatments, we need to always be thinking: how does this compare to doing nothing? (We usually call this 'monitoring the patient'). Now we look at different natural histories in turn.

Spontaneously remitting illnesses

The typical time-course of a spontaneously remitting illness is shown in Figure 5.3. Time is on the horizontal axis, and the severity of illness on the vertical axis. Notice that even if we do nothing the disease will get better with time: 'cure' occurs naturally. Any benefit of treatment comes from either reducing the time to 'cure' or to relieving the severity of symptoms, while nature takes its course; it does not influence whether the patient gets better or not. We therefore need to be particularly careful about the potential harms of treatment.

Returning to Case 2 from Box 5.1:

> Georgina Playford (aged 7) presents with a scaly rash. It started about a week ago, and spread alarmingly across her body over the course of a day (Figure 5.4). Her mother admits to noticing one spot that appeared first when questioned about this specifically. It preceded the main rash by several days, but didn't think it was important. The rash is not itchy, but her mother is worried about its appearance. She is worried she will transmit something infectious to other children at home (and at school).

This clinical pattern is typical of *Pityriasis rosacea*, an illness of unknown aetiology, which is reasonably common (GPs see a case about every 6 months). The features that point to the diagnoses are:

> Typical diagnostic features of *Pityriasis rosacea* include: one symptom only (red scaly spots); variable number of spots; scales face inwards (suggestive of ruptured shallow blisters); spots are aligned along dermatomes; the trunk is affected more than limbs; pruritus (itching) in less than 10%; preceding 'herald spot'. The natural history for the condition is to resolve spontaneously in about 2–3 months.

Pityriasis rosacea is unusual in having only one set of symptoms (spots – that are quantifiable). Moreover there is no evidence of any effective treatment. This makes it an ideal simplified model. We can picture the course of the illness. It enables us to imagine how the illness varies from person to person. Sometimes there are many more spots than others (the severity of symptoms is very variable). The symptoms last longer or shorter in different episodes of illness (the time-course of symptoms is also variable, although rather less so) (see Figure 5.5).

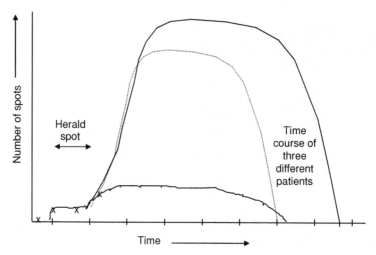

Figure 5.6 Extrapolating from the previous trajectory of the illness history to set out prognosis possibilities.

This way of illustrating the illness (Figure 5.6) enables us to picture one important characteristic of the illness for our patient: provide a prognosis.

> Georgina: *'No doctor, I have never heard of Pityriasis rosea. Is it dangerous? Do I need some treatment? Can I give it to Henry? What's going to happen? This looks just awful!'*

Pityriasis rosea is unusual in having a very predictable time course. Following a week or so of the herald lesion (which is not always noticed by the patient) the spots appear rapidly. They last from 6 to 8 weeks and then fade away (Figure 5.6). A few people need some help with the itching, but most are simply concerned about the appearance of the spots, and what they mean.

Estimating the individual's prognosis requires several steps, some of them simultaneously: deciding the severity of the illness (from the number of spots in this case), and then the likely duration of the illness to date. Then one can extrapolate forward in time to estimate the likely time of resolution of the illness. The process usually requires the taking of history to plot imaginary points on the possible illness trajectories.

For Georgina's spots it has to be estimated where on the illness trajectory she now lies, and whether she has a serious illness (many spots) or whether she has simply advanced along it a long way (Figure 5.6).

With *Pityriasis rosea* there is no effective treatment. There is no need for treatment because spontaneous remitting illnesses resolve by definition. But when a treatment is available, then the management options become more complicated.

Recurrent intermittent disease

Spontaneously remitting conditions may sometimes recur, and hence be considered as recurrent or intermittent conditions. Individual episodes follow the same model and principles as the spontaneously remitting disease. The crucial extra dimension is the likelihood or frequency of recurrence. Hence when describing to a patient the prognosis during a first episode, we would need to let them know about the natural history of this episode (as with spontaneously remitting disease) and about the chance and frequency of recurrence. For example, a patient after their first episode of renal colic or gout will be interested to know about the chances of a recurrence.

Consider Case 3 (from Box 5.1):

> A 50-year-old statistician has recently had an episode of renal colic. After a few weeks of intermittent pain, he passed a small calculus (kidney stone), much to his relief. He is now feeling fine but is worried about the chance of it happening again.

What can you tell him? We might get away with just saying something vague such as that they 'sometimes' recur. But this patient is a statistician, and wants some better quantification. First of all, the lifetime risk of having a renal calculus is around 10%. So that gives a starting point. Even if he had never had a stone there is 'some' chance that he will have one. But presumably his chance is higher, given he has had one episode.

Where would we get such information? The ideal source of data would be what is called an inception cohort study: a representative group of patients followed with their first episode of renal colic. We would like to know if anything modified the chances of recurrence also. Does age, or the size or type of stone change the probabilities? One way to find such information would be from textbooks (but unfortunately the couple on my shelf did not provide it). If that fails or the answer in the textbooks is unreferenced or vague, then you might check for prognostic studies by going to *PubMed: Clinical Queries*. But this is straying into the processes of evidence-based practice, and we refer the reader on to other sources for that.

The pattern of recurrences will usually be randomly scattered. However, random patterns are not even patterns (so that, for example, an attack every 4 weeks is not random). Random patterns often appear to be clumped in some way, and can easily lead to inappropriate inferences about triggers.

Chronic (non-progressive) illness

A chronic disease is a long-term condition in which the manifestations never fully disappear. Fluctuations may occur, and in fact are the usual pattern. Because of the ageing of the population and the increasing burden of disease due to lifestyle factors, such as poor diet and lack of exercise, the proportion of disease that fits this pattern is now much greater than in the past. Many chronic diseases show fluctuation around a slow deterioration in symptoms over time.

For example, many degenerative diseases fit this pattern. Degenerative diseases are progressive conditions for which we would all be headed if we lived long enough. Most of our organs would eventually 'fail', and our main hope is for our organs to outlive us. Renal function, lung function, vascular function, skin resilience, glucose tolerance and sensory functions all deteriorate with time, but at different rates for different people. Once a critical threshold of function is reached, we become symptomatic, and in particular are susceptible to the temporary deficits or strains induced by other diseases. For example, a chest infection that would only slow down a healthy person might be life threatening in someone with heart failure.

Because of the nature of chronic disease, the focus of management is on control and not cure. Monitoring is an important element of this. Patients need to be made aware and come to accept the long-term nature of the disease, and be actively involved in their own management.

Because of their long-term focus on a single disease, patients can often come to know more about the disease than their doctors. Rather than feel intimidated, we can see this as a benefit and that mutual learning may occur.

The fluctuations of such conditions generally mean we will see the patient during times when their symptoms have recently worsened. Fortunately, 'regression to the mean' will mean that such flares are likely to settle even with no treatment. Decisions to start more aggressive treatment need to be tempered by this knowledge of the likely natural history. A danger with such regression to the mean is that both patient and clinician may come to false inferences about the benefits of particular treatments. If you suspect this, then using a diary and setting up an informal crossover trial may be a reasonable course (see Chapter 7 on Monitoring).

A main aim of treatment for degenerative conditions is to slow the rate of progression. For example, renal failure may be slowed by good control of blood pressure; COPD may be slowed by cessation of smoking; and peripheral neuropathy may be slowed by better diabetic control.

Progressive diseases

The natural history of some illnesses, notably most cancers, is one of relentless progress. As with other patterns, an understanding of the natural history is important for informing the patient and for treatment decisions. The rate of progression is crucial: will this be rapid or slow?

Patients often assume that almost all cancers are relentlessly progressive. This is not always the case, and particularly with screen-detected cancers. We need to make certain that patients have a realistic understanding of the likely progress of their particular disease.

When a disease is rapidly progressive, doctors and their patients will often attempt treatments with potentially severe side effects, such as radical surgery, in the hope of a cure. In some cases, early treatment may be vital. As always, we need to weigh up the possible benefits and harms of treatment versus the natural history of the disease. In particular, we may need to try to predict

Table 5.2 Different types of prognostic factors.

Type of factor	Detail	Example
Independent of the disease process	The factor is related to general health more than the disease itself	Age for ischaemic heart disease
Dependant on the disease process	These are understood in terms of the disease mechanisms	Presence of estrogen receptors in breast cancers
Risk factors	Influence whether the individual will be susceptible to disease at all	Being female or developing Systemic Lupus Erythematosus

individual variation in progression rate. Recall Gould's mesothelioma, which had a much better prognosis than average.

Prognosis: an altered natural history

The natural history may of course be altered (hopefully improved!), by appropriate treatment. Prognosis is the history with treatment, so that when we say *the prognosis for childhood leukaemia was poor but is now much better*, we mean that the (untreated) natural history is poor, as was the case in the past, but that modern treatment improves this greatly.

Prognostic factors
In addition to treatment, many other factors can help predict the likely course of illness. These are called prognostic factors. Sometimes they are independent of the disease process (such as age); sometimes dependent (such as the severity or stage of the illness); or there may be risk factors for getting the disease (such as being female for developing Systemic Lupus Erythematosus) (see Table 5.2).

Managing expectations
Informing the patient of the natural history is an essential first part of informed choice about treatment. A conversation with a young patient about a shingles on his abdomen might go like this:

'Yes Frank, this is clearly shingles. Have you heard of it?'
Frank: *'Not really doctor. I think a friend of my Mum's had it a long time ago, and was very sick in some way...'*
'It's caused by a virus in a single nerve. It may get a little worse in the area it currently covers, but won't spread to other parts of your body. In young folk it's usually gone in about 2 weeks.'
Frank: *'OK. But can't it cause really bad, long-lasting pain?'*

'Yes that can occur, but almost never in a person as young as you; it really only happens to people over 50, and even then relatively uncommon. The only risk I do need to warn you about is that, while the lesions are active, you can transmit chickenpox and that is dangerous for pregnant women. Are any of your friends or contacts potentially pregnant?'

Frank: *'My sister-in-law is pregnant, but I haven't seen her recently. How long should I avoid contact?'*

Doctor: *'Just until the lesions are inactive. So when you've had no new lesions, and the old ones look like they are healing, you'd be safe again...'*

Offering a prognosis must be done carefully. It is easy to damage the clinician's credibility by being wrong. Let us imagine Case 2 (Box 5.1) 7 weeks later.

Georgina's mother: *'Doctor, I thought you said this rash would be gone by now! Do you think it is time Georgina I was referred to a dermatologist?'*

It sounds as if the clinician was over-optimistic. This is a mistake rarely made by astute doctors in the past. If anything they were pessimistic with prognoses, so that patients were more likely to receive a happy surprise. It would have been better to give the least optimistic prognosis.

Perhaps we should learn a lesson from this when we give women an estimated date of delivery (EDD) early in pregnancy. We (the medical profession, based on what is likely to cause problems to foetal-maternal health) had defined a normal date of delivery as anywhere in the month straddling the EDD. But the EDD often becomes over-emphasised in a woman's mind, especially if she has had enough of being pregnant. So often obstetric services are nagged by women wanting to be induced because the EDD has passed... Perhaps we should say something different.

'So, Angela, my estimate of when you will have the baby is any time in the month before April 3rd next year.'*

Further reading

Dunn S. *Survival Curves: The Basics* (http://www.cancerguide.org/scurve_basic.html).

---

* This being EDD + 2 weeks.

CHAPTER 6

Making clinical management decisions

As any doctor knows, it is not possible to practice medicine from a protocol or an algorithm, or even from evidence-based guidelines. We need guidelines that outline the best evidence for the potential harms and benefits of treatment, but clinical management decisions are complex and incorporate many factors that are not easily incorporated into protocols or guidelines. We need to be able to integrate the evidence with many other factors, such as the patient's values and objectives.

As we discussed in the introduction, doctors primarily use an approach to clinical decision making that is perhaps best described by the recognition primed decision-making model.[6] They recognise that a clinical situation fits a particular pattern, and based on this make management decisions. They are often not conscious of making decisions, but act in response to the pattern of the situation in front of them.

This approach to clinical problem solving, however, does not explain how to incorporate new evidence into the decision-making process, or how to apply evidence from the groups of patients in trials to the individual patient in front of you, or how to incorporate the patient's values and objectives into the decision-making process.

We also outlined the Pro-Act-Ive approach to health care decision making, that is, a formal approach for explicitly laying out all the alternatives, considering the consequences of the alternatives, weighing up the relative merits of each alternative and choosing the option that results in the greatest net benefit. In this chapter we will illustrate the use of the Pro-Act-Ive framework to make a decision regarding treatment. We will use a clinical case to demonstrate how you could, with enough time and resources, explicitly work through a clinical decision using this framework. As you will see as we work through the case, however, that what at first appears to be a relatively straightforward decision can rapidly become highly complex. It would be extremely time-consuming and laborious to attempt to make clinical decisions in this way. However, it is worthwhile to understand the principles of this approach and to be able to adapt it for more everyday use.

Box 6.1 Madison's Story

It is Monday morning in your general practice in the suburbs. The nurses have asked you to see a sick child as an add-on to your booked appointments.

Madison is a 22-month-old girl who has been unwell for the past 48 hours. She has been unhappy, crying occasionally, has a fever, is not eating or drinking well and is waking up and crying several times through the night. She has two older siblings, who are at primary school and are well. Both her parents work full-time and she goes to a child-care centre near her mother's work on weekdays. Madison has generally been a well child, but she had a similar episode about 6 months ago that took a week to resolve. Her immunisation is up-to-date. On examination, she is not dehydrated, her temperature is 37.9°C and the only abnormality of note is a right dull red tympanic membrane.

PRO – defining the problem and the objectives

P = defining the problem

Madison appears to have acute otitis media (see Box 6.1). This may be due to either viral or bacterial causes. Antibiotics may be of benefit in treating bacterial infections and may lessen the risk of severe complications that might occur with bacterial infections.

R = reframe the problem from multiple perspectives

The most immediate problem is to ensure that Madison is not suffering any immediate severe or potentially life-threatening complications, such as meningitis, pneumonia or dehydration. Once you have established that there is no sign of these complications, you need to consider all the other potential perspectives to this problem. Madison is obviously distressed and is in pain, so you would like to do something to alleviate this. She is not sleeping well, which is disrupting all the family and which her parents find particularly distressing. Her mother works casually and so will not be paid if she needs to stay home and look after Madison, but she will still need to pay child-care fees. Her mother is worried that this is the second episode in 6 months and that Madison is going to have recurrent episodes. Her mother is also worried that these episodes may be harming Madison's hearing and language development. Finally, she wants to make sure that her other children do not get the same illness.

As the general practitioner looking after this child, you are aware that acute otitis media is generally a self-limiting illness, but there is a very small risk of complications such as meningitis and mastoiditis. The acute episode may be followed by chronic otitis media, which will generally be asymptomatic but can cause some temporary hearing loss. You are aware that many parents will expect antibiotics for their child's ear infections, but are also aware that this is causing a major public health problem due to increasing antibiotic resistance.

O = focus on the objectives

After discussion with Madison's mother, there seem to be a number of priorities:

1 Minimise the severity of Madison's symptoms, particularly the pain (and consequent sleep disturbance).
2 Minimise the duration of her illness.
3 Reduce the risk of complications, particularly meningitis, mastoiditis and chronic otitis media with any associated short- or long-term hearing problems or language delay.
4 Reduce the risk of spread of the illness to other family members.
5 Reduce the use of antibiotics in order to reduce the future risk of antibiotic resistance.

Act – determining the alternatives, consequences and trade-offs

A = consider all relevant alternatives

Once we have determined the potential objectives of treatment, we need to consider our alternatives for treatment. These are:

1 Do nothing. This is a potential course of action and it is useful as a baseline to compare doing nothing with the potential harms and benefits of other treatments. It is unlikely that you will want to do nothing in this case, however, as Madison is in pain and you will probably want to do something to relieve this.
2 Provide pain relief.
3 Provide an antibiotic; or,
4 provide a prescription for an antibiotic and ask Madison's mother to only fill the prescription if she does not get better within a few days.

Providing pain relief may be considered as an alternative on its own or may be combined with option 3 or 4.

In addition to these immediate alternatives, you will also need to make decisions regarding what to advise the mother on what warning signs should cause her to return and if you need to review the child again at a later date.

C = consider the consequences of each alternative and estimate the chances

What are the chances that each of the alternatives above can help meet the objectives that you have set?

It is at this point that we need to consider the clinical evidence. We need to consider the evidence for the impact of each alternative on each of the objectives and how this evidence might apply to Madison. Much of the emphasis in the teaching of evidence-based medicine has been on how to search for evidence for clinical questions and how to determine the validity of that evidence. There has been less focus on the application of the evidence to individuals and to the integration of the evidence with values. The five steps of evidence-based medicine are:

1 to ask a focussed clinical question;
2 to search for the evidence;
3 to appraise the evidence;
4 to apply the evidence to the individual patient;
5 to evaluate the process.

Step 1: Ask a focussed clinical question

We have defined our clinical question through the characteristics of the case and the defining of our objectives. Because we are considering a number of objectives of treatment and a number of alternative treatments, we have a series of clinical questions. As an example we have:

What is the effect of antibiotics (intervention) compared with doing nothing (comparator) on pain (outcome) in a 2-year-old with acute otitis media (patient)?

We need to consider the effect of each of the alternative treatments on each of the objectives. It is helpful to try and define our clinical question in this format:

P (patient)
I (intervention)
C (comparator), and
O (outcome)

Step 2: Search for the evidence

Searching for the best evidence to answer a clinical question can be complex. The best evidence would be a systematic review of a number of randomised controlled trials in the relevant population. It may be possible to find such a review on *Medline*, the largest database of published medical literature published by the National Library of Medicine in the United States.[78] For systematic reviews of the effectiveness of health care intervention, the largest database is the *Cochrane Library*, published by Wileys.[79] There are now also many other sources of information that bring together clinical research on particular topics, for example '*Clinical Evidence*', published by BMJ Publishing,[80] or '*UpToDate*'.[81]

There has been a *Cochrane Review* on the effectiveness of antibiotics for the treatment of acute otitis media.[82]

Step 3: Appraising the evidence

The ability to critically appraise clinical research is now seen as a core skill for all the clinical disciplines. There are many excellent textbooks on this topic.[83–86]

We will not try to summarise all the details of the skills that are necessary to critically appraise clinical research here. For estimates on the effectiveness of treatment as in the case here, however, the most valid evidence comes from randomised controlled trials. If trials are well designed, they minimise the potential biases that might affect estimates of effectiveness. The results of trials can be combined together in a meta-analysis, a statistical technique for synthesising the results from a number of trials. A well-designed meta-analysis, conducted as part of a systematic review that looks for all the potential evidence in an area, gives the most accurate and precise estimates of the effectiveness of an intervention. We are fortunate that for this clinical question there have been a number of trials and the trials have been combined in a meta-analysis (see Box 6.2).

Step 4: Apply the evidence to the individual patient
This is one of the most difficult steps and least understood parts off the evidence-based medicine process. Again, we can think of the process as being in a number of stages:
(a) determine the possible beneficial and harmful effects of treatment;
(b) determine if there is a predictable variation in the relative effects of treatment between sub-groups of patients;
(c) examine if effects vary with risk level;
(d) estimate the predicted benefits and harms for an individual patient (in terms of absolute risk changes).
We will use the results of the *Cochrane Review* of the effects of antibiotics for acute otitis media (see Box 6.2) to illustrate how we can apply evidence to the individual patient.

From the information in this abstract, we can begin to estimate the consequences of the alternatives above.

(a) *Determine the possible beneficial and harmful effects of treatment.* Antibiotics do not appear to have any effect on the pain or distress of acute otitis media at 24 hours, but there is some reduction in the number of children suffering pain at 2 to 7 days. On the basis of the results of these trials, we can predict that if we see 100 children with acute otitis media, 21 will still have pain at 2 to 7 days if they are not treated with antibiotics. If we treated all 100 children with antibiotics, 14 will still have pain at 2 to 7 days (an absolute reduction of 7 in 100 children or 7%). We can show the same numbers pictorially (see Figure 6.1). Therefore, there is some benefit from treating acute otitis media with antibiotics in terms of reducing pain in the medium term.

The most commonly reported effect from trials is the relative risk or the relative risk reduction or the odds ratio. The relative risk and odds ratio can be thought of as measuring much the same effect and will generally give similar results, particularly if the risk of the event that you are looking at is relatively uncommon, say less than about 20%. The methods for calculating

Box 6.2 Some Evidence for Antibiotics for Sore Throat[82]

Glasziou PP, Del Mar CB, Sanders SL, Hayem M. Antibiotics for acute otitis media in children.[82]

ABSTRACT

Background
Acute otitis media is one of the most common diseases in early infancy and childhood. Antibiotic use for acute otitis media varies from 31% in the Netherlands to 98% in the USA and Australia.

Objectives
The objective of this review was to assess the effects of antibiotics for children with acute otitis media.

Search Strategy
We searched the *Cochrane Controlled Trials Register*, MEDLINE, *Index Medicus* (pre-1965), Current Contents and reference lists of articles from 1958 to January 2000. The search was updated in March 2003.

Selection Criteria
Randomised trials comparing antimicrobial drugs with placebo in children with acute otitis media.

Data collection and analysis
Three reviewers independently assessed trial quality and extracted data.

Main Results
Ten trials were eligible but only seven trials, with a total of 2,202 children, included patient-relevant outcomes. The methodological quality of the included trials was generally high. All trials were from developed countries. The trials showed no reduction in pain at 24 hours, but a 30% relative reduction (95% confidence interval 19% to 40%) in pain at two to seven days. Since approximately 80% of patients will have settled spontaneously in this time, this means an absolute reduction of 7% or that about 15 children must be treated with antibiotics to prevent one child having some pain after two days. There was no effect of antibiotics on hearing problems of acute otitis media, as measured by subsequent tympanometry. However, audiometry was done in only two studies and incompletely reported. Nor did antibiotics influence other complications or recurrence. There were few serious complications seen in these trials: only one case of mastoiditis occurred in a penicillin treated group.

Reviewers' conclusions
Antibiotics provide a small benefit for acute otitis media in children. As most cases will resolve spontaneously, this benefit must be weighed against the possible adverse reactions. Antibiotic treatment may play an important role in reducing the risk of mastoiditis in populations where it is more common.

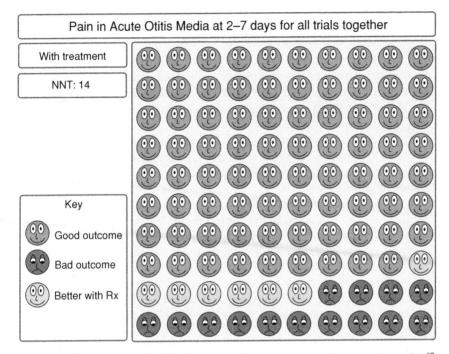

Figure 6.1 The risk of pain at 2 to 7 days in children treated with acute otitis media.[87] Reproduced from http://www.nntonline.net, with permission from Dr Chris Cates.

relative risk, relative risk reduction and absolute risk reduction are shown in Box 6.3.

Table 6.1 provides data for other outcomes reported in the trials. Based on the results from these trials, antibiotics had no effect on the risk of recurrence, ear perforation, abnormal hearing at 1 or 3 months or the risk of otitis media in the other ear. Because mastoiditis, meningitis and other sequelae of acute otitis media are relatively rare in the settings of these trials, the trials were not large enough to detect any possible difference in these outcomes between the children treated with antibiotics and the children treated with symptoms. Of the 2,202 children in these trials, one child developed mastoiditis, and that was in a child who had been treated with penicillin. Because trials cannot be large enough to detect a difference in rare events, such as mastoiditis, we may need to use other types of data to be certain about the effect of antibiotics on these types of events. For example, a time series analysis has shown that there has been no increase in the rate of admission for mastoiditis following the decline in the use of antibiotics for respiratory tract infections.[88]

As well as the benefits of treatment, we need to consider if there are any potential harms of treatment. The potential harms of using antibiotics are the side effects of the antibiotics (vomiting, diarrhoea or allergic reaction) and the wider public health problem of increasing antibiotic resistance. The data from

---

Box 6.3 Relative Risk, Relative Risk Reduction, Absolute Risk Reduction and Number Needed to Treat

The *relative risk* is the risk of an event in the intervention group divided by the risk of an event in the control group. In this case, it is the risk of pain at two to seven days in the group treated with antibiotics divided by the risk of pain in the group treated with placebo. From the graph above, this is equal to $14/100 \div 21/100 = 67\%$.

The *relative risk reduction* is 1 minus the relative risk. In this case, it is $100\% - 67\% = 33\%$. In the abstract above, it states that the relative risk reduction for pain at two to seven days was 30%. The difference is due to minor rounding errors.

The *absolute risk reduction* is the risk of an event in the intervention group minus the risk of an event in the control group. For pain at two to seven days, this is equal to 21% minus 14% = 7%.

Another way of expressing the clinical value is the *number needed to treat* (equal to the inverse of the absolute risk reduction). If the absolute risk reduction for pain at two to seven days was 7%, the number needed to treat is $100/7 = 14$. That is, we would need to treat 14 children with antibiotics in order to prevent one child still having pain at two to seven days.

The relative risk reduction will generally be larger than the absolute risk reduction, but the size of the absolute risk reduction provides a better indication of the clinical value of a treatment.

Table 6.1 Results of the meta-analysis of trials on the benefits of antibiotics for treating acute otitis media.[82]

Outcome	Relative effect (RR or OR)	Absolute effect (NNT)	Is the result statistically significant?
Pain/distress			
24 hours	1.03		Not significant
2–7 days	0.70	14	Significant
Recurrence	1.00		
Perforation	0.51		Not significant
Abnormal hearing test (tympanometry)			
1 month	0.91		Not significant
3 months	0.75		Not significant
Contralateral OM	0.45		Not significant

Table 6.2 Results of the meta-analysis of trials on the harms of antibiotics for treating acute otitis media.

Outcome	Relative effect (RR or OR)	Absolute effect (Number needed to harm)	Is the result statistically significant?
Vomiting or diarrhoea or rash	1.97	17	Significant

the trials included in the meta-analysis on the risk of vomiting, diarrhoea or rash are given in Table 6.2.

This means that for every 17 children that we treat with antibiotics for acute otitis media, one extra child will develop vomiting, diarrhoea or a rash (compared with children treated with a placebo). Again, because of the rarity of the event, no child in these trials suffered an anaphylactic reaction. It is also not possible to measure the risk of increasing antibiotic resistance from these trials.

(b) *Determine if there is a predictable variation in the relative effects of treatment between sub-groups of patients.* It may be that some groups of patients receive more or less benefit from the treatment than others. We need to base our treatment decisions on what we know about the effectiveness of treatment in a group of patients, as this is the only way that we can test and estimate the true size of the effect. What we can never predict is the exact probability of the benefit for the individual patient sitting in front of us. What may be possible, however, is to determine the size of the effect in a particular sub-group of patients (based on the data from the trials) or it may be possible to predict the effect for certain types of patients will be possibly greater or less than that seen in the overall result in the trials.

Two of the trials included in the review showed that benefits were greatest in younger children (less than 2 years old) and in children with bilateral acute otitis media. In one of the trials included in the review, a sub-group analysis was conducted to determine which groups of children benefited most from antibiotic treatment. This analysis showed that children who presented with high fevers and vomiting benefited most.

In most of the trials that were included in this review, a certain proportion of children were excluded from entering the trials because they were considered by the treating physician to be 'too sick'. How this was defined varied slightly between the trials, but it is important that we remember that we cannot generalise from the results of these trials to the treatment of children who are seriously unwell.

Certain factors about the patient may alter the potential harms and benefits of treatment. Often doctors assume that factors such as age, gender and other demographic or biological factors influence the benefits of treatment. In this case, the age of the child is a factor, but such biological factors do not necessarily modify the effects of treatment. More likely modifiers are factors such as the severity or duration of the illness and whether the disease is a recurrence or not. It may be that in the future we will be able to do genetic testing, which will be able to better predict who will benefit from certain treatments.

(c) *Examine if effects vary with risk level.* One of the main justifications for using antibiotics to treat acute otitis media in the past was to avoid the potentially serious complications, such as mastoiditis or meningitis. These are now uncommon complications in metropolitan regions of developed countries. The potential harms from routine antibiotic usage are unlikely to offset the potential benefits of preventing complications that occur only very rarely. There are regions, however, where such complications remain common. For example, the risk of severe complications from acute otitis media is much higher in indigenous communities in Australia. In these populations, the benefits of routine antibiotic treatment for acute otitis media are likely to be much greater than in the general population.

We may also be able to test how the benefit of treatment changes with the underlying risk of an event. Commonly, the relative benefit of treatment (measured by the relative risk or relative risk reduction) stays relatively constant, not varying with the underlying risk of the patient. This means that patients at high risk of an event gain more than patients at low risk of an event.

For example, it is known that aspirin helps to reduce the risk of myocardial infarction. However, it has a greater benefit in patients who are at a high risk of an event (for example, patients who have already had a myocardial infarction) than in patients who are low risk (for example, patients who have previously been healthy). The risk of the most important complication of aspirin, gastrointestinal bleeding, is not related to the risk of a myocardial infarction. The benefits of treatment are likely to outweigh the possible risk of gastro-intestinal bleeding in patients at a high risk of myocardial infarction, but not necessarily in patients at low risk.

We can investigate how the risk varies with the underlying risk of an event by drawing a L'Abbé plot of the results of the trials included in the meta-analysis of randomised controlled trials of antibiotics for acute otitis media (see Figure 6.2). This graph shows the risk of an event on the horizontal axis and the risk of an event in the experimental group on the vertical axis. If the risk is the same in both groups (that is, there is no overall treatment effect), the trial will lie on the line of equality from the origin (indicating a relative risk of 1). The further a trial lies below the line of equality, the greater the estimated treatment effect (the distance between the trial and the line of equality is a measure of the absolute risk difference). The size of each of the trials can be indicated by the size of the bubble.

In the trials of antibiotics to treat acute otitis media, the size of the absolute treatment effect (the absolute risk difference), appears to get larger as the risk of an event in the trial population (indicated by the distance along the horizontal axis) gets larger. The trials lie roughly along a straight line from the origin. This implies a constant relative risk (the relative relationship between the risk of an event in the intervention group and the control group stays

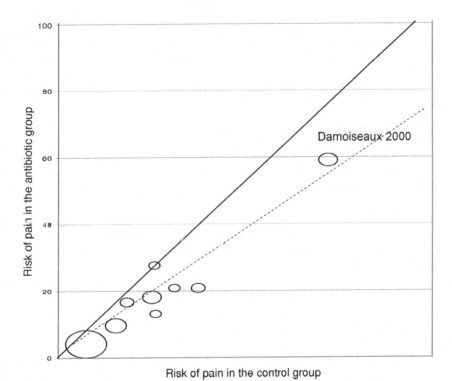

Figure 6.2 L'Abbé plot of antibiotics for pain for acute otitis media at 2–7 days.

constant). This confirms our belief that the benefits of antibiotics are likely to increase in populations at a high risk of events.

This graph (see Figure 6.2) also highlights a further point. The risk of pain at two to seven days is much higher in the trial labelled Damoiseaux, and is almost 80%. This trial was a trial of amoxicillin versus placebo in children aged under 2 years.[85] It may be worth exploring why the risk of pain at two to seven days was so much greater in this trial than in previous trials.

(d) *Estimate the predicted benefits and harms for an individual patient (in terms of absolute risk changes).* Madison is a 2-year-old child. She is therefore in an age group that is more likely to benefit from treatment than will all children who suffer from acute otitis media. However, she does not have a very high fever, vomiting or bilateral acute otitis media, which are other indicators of increased treatment benefit.

T = identify and estimate the trade-offs

Based on the best evidence that we have available, providing an antibiotic will possibly shorten the duration of the illness, but increases the risk of side effects such as vomiting and diarrhoea. It also carries the risk to public health by increasing the risk of antibiotic resistance. There do not appear to be any long-term benefits of antibiotics in terms of preventing the possible complications of the disease.

If the treatment of pain was the only objective in this case, we might consider offering analgesia rather than an antibiotic. If appears that antibiotics may offer some marginal benefit in shortening the duration of the illness as measured by symptoms. This needs to be traded off against the potential harms, such as the adverse effects and increasing antibiotic resistance.

IVE – integration and exploration

I = Integrate the evidence and the values

Now that we have considered all the potential consequences of each alternative, we need to integrate all the available evidence and the values that we place on each of the outcomes. In this case, the evidence for the difference between treating with antibiotics and treating with analgesia is rather small and almost offset by the potential harms of using an antibiotic. There may be some small benefit in terms of the duration of the illness, particularly in children younger than 2 years of age. This small benefit may be of importance in this particular case. Overall, there is no clear answer in this case and it may be that it depends on the values of the mother, which is the best course of action.

V = optimise the expected Value

In this case, there is no alternative that is clearly optimal. Based on the research literature, the potential harms and benefits of treatment are quite close. It is therefore difficult to say which alternative gives the greatest expected value. We will probably want to prescribe antibiotics to some children, and it appears that the children that are most likely to benefit are those under 2 years and those who have signs of being more seriously unwell, for example with a high fever. In this case, Madison is less than 2 years old, but does not have a high fever. Again, it is not clear which is the best decision for this case. One alternative that has become popular is to provide the parent with an antibiotic prescription, but advise them only to use it if the child does not get better in a few days. This is not entirely logical, in that the benefit of antibiotics is not related to the duration of the illness, but it does reduce the rate of antibiotic prescribing.

E = Explore the assumptions and evaluate uncertainty

When there is a decision that has serious consequences and particularly when we will need to make the decision recurrently, or the decision will last for a long time, it is also important to examine how certain we are about our estimates of harm and benefit and how variation around these estimates might affect our decision. In decision theory, this is called sensitivity analysis. We particularly need to think through all the potential consequences of our decision making.

Decision regret and clinical decision making

Both patients and doctors tend to be relatively risk averse. That is, we try to protect ourselves from risky decisions. We are particularly aware of potential risks involved with treatments and try to avoid high-risk treatments and procedures. If the alternative is almost certainly death, however, both doctors and patients will often choose high-risk procedures, such as radical surgery or stem cell transplants, even if the odds of cure from such treatments may be low.

In the case described above, however, the more risky option is to do nothing. We are likely to feel extremely responsible if we do not treat a child with antibiotics and they develop some severe complication of the infection. This will weigh on us much more heavily than the harm we to do to potentially many more individuals by increasing antibiotic resistance. There is, therefore, a natural bias to prescribing antibiotics in a greater proportion of cases than the evidence would suggest.

Bringing clinical decision making back to the real world

As you can see, a clinical decision that happens in countless surgeries around the world every day is in fact extremely complex. It would be impossible to work through the Pro-Act-Ive sort of decision-making model for every clinical situation. Having seen the evidence and worked through this approach once, however, we are now be able to summarise our clinical decision into some simple heuristics:

1 Overall there are few short-term benefits and no apparent long-term benefits from prescribing antibiotics for acute otitis media. This is a potential for serious long-term harm, through increasing antibiotic resistance. It is therefore not wise to prescribe antibiotics to all children with acute otitis media.

2 Analgesia may be able to provide the same short-term benefits with fewer potential harms of treatment.

3 There are some children who will receive greater benefit from antibiotic treatment. These are children who are at particularly high risk of complications, for example indigenous children, younger children and children who present with severe symptoms. It may therefore be best to restrict antibiotics to children in these categories.

By examining the clinical evidence and the potential consequences of each of the alternatives, we can reduce our clinical decision making to something much more manageable and able to be used in the everyday clinical setting.

CHAPTER 7
Monitoring in chronic disease

Know which abnormality you are going to follow during treatment. Pick something you can measure.

Clifton Meador, *A Little Book of Doctors' Rules*[52]

Monitoring is a common clinical activity, particularly in primary and ambulatory care. It comprises between a third and half of all tests ordered in primary care and outpatients, and there is additional home monitoring undertaken by patients. Yet, it is surprisingly understudied, and poorly understood, compared to therapy or diagnosis.[89]

The essence of monitoring of a chronic or recurrent condition is periodic measurement followed by adjustment of the management. This monitoring and adjustment is what makes up most of the routine visits for long-term conditions. We have to choose several things:
• what measurements to monitor
• how often to measure and check
• decide when is control inadequate and then
• how to adjust treatment.

How do we choose? There are several important principles we will cover that assists in answering these questions for each condition. However, there are also several common errors of monitoring to avoid:
• re-checking too soon
• over-reacting to chance fluctuations
• over-adjusting therapy.

The aim of course is to achieve the best possible control with the minimum of monitoring effort.

Why is monitoring important?

Poor choices in each element can lead to poor control, inefficient use of time and resources and dangerous adjustments to treatment. For example, an audit of serum digoxin monitoring in one UK teaching hospital found that the logic behind more than 80% of the tests requested could not be established, the timing of tests reflected poor understanding of the clinical pharmacokinetics and about one result in four was followed by an inappropriate clinical decision. Improvements are possible. For example, a computerised reminder of inappropriate testing reduced the volume of anti-epileptic drug concentration monitoring by 20%,[90] a decision support system for anticoagulation with

Box 7.1 Examples of Chronic Diseases Caused by Loss of Control

Chronic disease	Physiological process for which control is impaired	Pathological effect
Hypothyroidism	Thyroid level	Too low
Diabetes	Insulin level	Too high
		Too variable
Renal failure	Serum K+	Too high
	Serum urea etc.	Too variable

warfarin led to an improvement from 45% to 63% of patients being within target range[91] and peak flow quality-control charts for asthmatics could detect exacerbations 4 days earlier than conventional methods.[92] Given the extent of monitoring, even modest improvements are likely to improve patient benefits and may reduce costs.

The purpose of monitoring

Why do we monitor? It is worth thinking about what a chronic disease is. The normal control of some physiological process has been lost so that the average, the fluctuation, or both, have become pathological (see Box 7.1). Monitoring (and adjustment of treatment) can be then thought of as a form of external homeostasis: bringing the average level and fluctuations back to more appropriate levels.

Should we monitor at all?

Though intuitively it seems obvious that monitoring is a good thing to do when managing chronic disease, we do not always do so or need to do so. For example, we use aspirin for preventing stroke *without* monitoring (or even measuring!) platelet aggregation. Sometimes our monitoring is so simple that we do not even think of it as monitoring; for example, in monitoring depression we often just ask if the patient is feeling better. Of course, this may be insufficient, and we may want to rethink our first question: what should we measure?

To decide if a condition is worth monitoring, each must be analysed on its own merits, estimating both the clinical effectiveness and opportunity cost of monitoring. Any patient benefit must be balanced against the downsides of monitoring (such as the inconvenience and costs, and the impact of false positive and false negative monitoring results that can lead to inappropriate or delayed actions). As with most other interventions, this ideally requires a randomised controlled trial. Benefits should be measured in terms of patient outcomes rather than the surrogate of time spent in a target range. However, few monitoring practices have undergone such trials.

For example, in a trial of drug monitoring in epilepsy, the monitored versus unmonitored patients were more often within control limits (8% versus 25%), but there was no change in the proportion remaining seizure free (38% versus 41%).[93] The surrogate measure was more optimistic than the more important patient-centred outcome.

Thinking about time

The consequences of the loss of internal control may be short-term, long-term, or both. Understanding this is critical on deciding how, and when, to monitor.

It is useful to ask three questions:
- What are the *short*-term consequences of loss of control?
- What are the *long*-term consequences of loss of control?
- Do *symptoms* give *early warning*?

For example, in insulin-dependent diabetes, extreme short-term fluctuations are sometimes common, and these may lead to catastrophic events with minimal prior warning (hypoglycemia – with loss of consciousness and threat to the viability of brain tissue, or hyperglycemia – with the threat of metabolic acidosis). Careful daily monitoring is needed.

In contrast, in hypercholesterolemia, cholesterol fluctuations do not lead to short-term consequences, even were they to be wide. Despite being asymptomatic, daily monitoring of cholesterol is unnecessary.

How does monitoring work?

The 'external homeostasis' of monitoring can be complex as it attempts to re-place the more complex physiological function of internal homeostasis. There are two broad parts:
- periodic measurement; and
- decisions about subsequent adjustment (which may be either clinician- or patient-controlled).

The improvements in care that arise from monitoring happen through several means:

1 *Altering treatments based on individual response.* For example replacing a hypertensive patient's antihypertensive with another because of either lack of response, or the appearance of unacceptable side-effects.

2 *Better titration of treatment.* For example increasing the dose of replacement thyroxin when the level of T4 and TSH in the blood indicate that the patient remains hypothyroid.

3 *Improvement of adherence.* For patients, in addition to using monitoring for providing an early signal for action, it may simply provide motivation to adhere to treatment. For example, patients are reminded to think about their diet when testing their blood sugars at home.

4 *Patients learning about non-treatment factors for better control.* For example, patients monitoring with a peak-flow meter can better appreciate that acute respiratory infections cause deterioration in their asthma (and offset deterioration by using their beta-agonist early).

Any formal evaluation of chronic disease monitoring effectiveness should be preceded by developmental work to understand these different functions. For example, a recent trial in which some diabetic patients were randomised to self-monitoring of risk factors showed a better achievement of target levels and a reduction in clinical events.[94] However, a randomised trial of the motivational effect of cholesterol measurement in UK general practice showed only a negligible benefit – a difference of 0.1mmol/l in total cholesterol.[95] The differences in the two findings may be attributable in part to differences in functions.

The need to decide how best to monitor is illustrated by a recent trial of three modes of peak flow monitoring in childhood asthma: no peak flow measurements (control), regular daily measurements, and monitoring only at times of symptoms. The latter group – children randomised to measure PEFR only when symptomatic – had lower asthma severity scores, fewer symptom days, and less health care utilization than children randomised to either daily peak flow monitoring or symptom-only monitoring.[96] The study illustrates that peak flow monitoring is helpful, but that the less intensive monitoring regimen is preferable.

The five phases of monitoring

The objective and methods of monitoring change over the course of treatment. There are five phases (see Table 7.1).

Control charts

Figure 7.1 illustrates a control chart for these five stages:
(a) We first *note the abnormal measurement* and begin a quick series of pre-treatment measurements to confirm the abnormal result;
(b) then, if appropriate, *initiate treatment* and monitor at short intervals to check response and achieve control;
(c) but *once control is achieved,* then
(d) the *intervals* may be longer, although may be supplemented by patient self-monitoring (small arrows);
(e) but when one measurement is more than 3 Standard Deviations (SDs) or 2 measurements are more than 2 SDs from target, we *adjust therapy* to re-establish control, and shorten the re-check interval; and, finally
(f) if treatment becomes unnecessary, a period of *post-cessation monitoring* may be required.

We now look at these phases in more detail.

1 *Pre-treatment monitoring.*   Pre-treatment monitoring should establish:
(a) the need for treatment;

Table 7.1 Objectives for the five phases of monitoring.

Phase		Monitoring objectives	Optimal interval
1	Pre-treatment	Check the need for treatment	*Short* – based on within person variability
		Establish a baseline for determining response and change	
2	Initial titration	Assess individual response to treatment	*Medium* – based on pharmacokinetics (e.g., drug half-life) and pharmaco-dynamics (physiological impact time) (wash-in)
		Assess immediate adverse effects	
		Achieve control	
3	Maintenance	Detect drift from control limits	*Long* – based on rate of random and systematic 'drift'
		Detect long-term harms	
4	Re-establish control	Bring level back within control limits.	Medium – see (2)
5	Cessation	Check safety of cessation	Medium – see (2)

(b) a baseline to judge the response to treatment or changes in the condition.
Generally we should not start treatment until we have sufficient measurements for a firm baseline. This firm baseline is needed to confirm that the degree of abnormality is beyond the initiation threshold. Serial measurements may 'normalise' before treatment for several reasons (see Box 7.2).

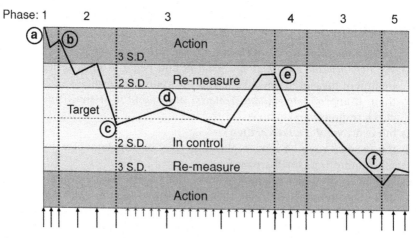

Figure 7.1 The five phases of treatment monitoring – large arrows are clinician measurements; small arrows are patient measurements. For numbers see text. From Glasziou et al.[89]

Box 7.2 Reasons for Normalisation of Serial Measurements

- Regression to the mean (the tendency of repeat tests to be closer to normal[97]) This is probably the most important reason
- Accommodation to measurement (e.g., with blood pressure measurement)
- Training effects (e.g., with peak flow meter)

For example, blood pressure falls as individuals get used to having it measured: in the first biennial check in the Framingham study the average blood pressure fell by 3.4 mmHg systolic and 2.4mmHg diastolic.[98]

Another example: among 99 Dutch patients with apparently raised blood pressure, re-measurement resulted in average reductions of 9mm Hg systolic and 4 mm Hg diastolic.[99] The same study suggested that two measurements were sufficient to establish the need for treatment in those well above the initiation threshold. For borderline patients even four measurements resulted in substantial misclassification.

2 *Initial titration: establishing response, control and safety.* Having established the need to start treatment, we should set a target and begin titration to achieve that target. However, achieving target is just one of several objectives of the initial titration phase, which should include:

- checking the individual's response to treatment,
- detecting unacceptable adverse effects,
- achieving the desired target range.

Monitoring during the early stages of therapy checks the response to treatment. That is, we are checking whether the therapy 'works' for this patient as expected on the basis of clinical trials in other patients. However, few patients are 'average' and hence predicting or checking their individual response is important. Sometimes an individual's response to treatment can be predicted by other measurements, such as their symptom pattern, their weight, or increasingly genetic testing (e.g., the dose requirement on initiating warfarin therapy is strongly related to a single CYP2C9 gene variants).[100] Sometimes it might be predicted by pharmacokinetic studies.

For example, in initiating tricyclic antidepressants, short-term measurement of the drug concentration can characterise individual metabolism and guide the long-term dose used.[101]

However, generally prediction is poor, and customising treatment usually requires some pragmatic trial-and-error. We can think of this phase as an 'n-of-1' trial establishing how well the treatment works.[102] Ideally, the estimate of effect will be based on both the measurements in that patient and the known effect from trials.[103]

During this phase the measurements should be more frequent than when the patient is fully controlled, but needs to allow for the full effect to be achieved. It may be helpful to ask patients to keep a diary during this period, to convince both you and them that there has been an adequate response. The diary needs to include the type of measure (see the Table at the end of this Chapter for some choices), the time of day and how frequently to measure.

The initiation phase should also be used to detect immediate or short-term adverse effects.[104] Hence, measures of potential harm should be assessed and monitored.

Almost half of the medicines in the electronic Medicines Compendium suggest some monitoring. Many drugs impact on renal function, and regular monitoring of creatinine and electrolytes is widely recommended.

A more specific example is clozapine therapy, for which weekly white cell counts are measured for the first few months to detect agranulocytosis, which occurs in 0.8% of patients.

However, the rationale for the timing of measurement is seldom explicit. The criteria for monitoring for adverse effects (similar to those for screening; see Chapter 8), include that:

- the effect is serious;
- there is a simple test;
- earlier detection is predictive, and
- change in treatment leads to a better outcome.[105]

3 *Monitoring during treatment.* Once a patient's measurements are close to the initial target, the objective of monitoring is to ensure that measurements stay within a reasonable range of that, the so-called '*control limits*'.

The control limits are set in order to ensure that we detect real changes in level while minimising false positives. These can come from:

- short-term measurement variability, or
- technical measurement error.

The degree of short-term variation may be estimated from population studies, sub-populations, or from the individual's own measurements. Because extreme measurements are unlikely to be due to short-term measurement variability, they may justify action to re-establish control.

One approach suggested by statistical control theory is to consider that a shift from control has occurred:[106]

- if a single measurement is outside a 3 standard deviation (SD) upper and lower control limit;
- if two or three successive measurements are more than 2 SD from the target.

Figure 7.1 shows these two sets of action thresholds; one for action ($\pm$3SD) and one for re-measurement ($\pm$2SD), with action if the repeat result is also more than 2 SD from the target.

Monitoring can be less frequent than during the initiation phase. The interval depends on the probability of being outside the control limits, which in turn depends on both random drift and systematic changes (progression or regression of disease).

The *measurements* intervals may be shorter than the *decision* interval at which the monitoring information is used to decide on whether control is adequate. For example, monitoring measurements of BP might be done daily by patients, but the decision point might be a monthly consultation at which the doctor looks at the average BP based on all measurements over the last month. This is illustrated in Figure 7.1, where multiple measures (3b – small arrows) occur between the decision points (3a – larger arrows). In some instances a single measurement will provide an assessment of average control over a period of weeks, e.g., HbA1C.

Ideally, a graphical presentation, such as a control chart, should be used to aid recording and deciding treatment changes (see Control Charts section below).

4 *Adjustment to re-establish control.* When we detect a clear drift beyond the control limits, we may alter management to re-establish control. As in the initiation phase, a shorter measurement interval is generally warranted until control is re-established.

This is difficult to do well. Audits have shown that clinical decisions taken as a result of monitoring are sub-optimal.

> For example, a New Zealand study of digoxin monitoring shows that 53% of ordered measurements were inappropriately timed, and that of the ordered measurements 5% led to inappropriate dose adjustments.[107]
>
> Patients too find this difficult: a survey of diabetes educators suggested that correct adjustment of insulin dose is the single hardest skill to teach.[108]

This is partly because of the lack of forethought – a planned and explicit response to different possible test results.

Furthermore, tests are seldom considered in context of past values, or in the knowledge of measurement variability. Instead, they usually arrive in isolation as a single value. To overcome this, we would suggest either providing patient-held records with a graphical display, or using medical record software that allows graphing over time, or preferably both.

5 *Cessation of treatment.* Most therapies are not life-long. To minimise unnecessary medications, we should have a clear stopping rule. Monitoring should provide information that informs whether, and when, to end therapy. Again, such decisions are usually based on a threshold level:

> **1** A negative outcome e.g., an adverse effect on renal function or frequency of epileptic seizures exceeding a threshold; or
>
> **2** A positive outcome (e.g., pain relief or blood pressure) falling below a minimum threshold.

However, the precise thresholds chosen and the monitoring interval depend on the phase of treatment. Cessation of treatment mirrors the first phases of pre-treatment and initiating treatment. A decision to stop based on current risks and control is made, treatment is withdrawn (perhaps in stages), and, after a 'wash-out' period (after which it is estimated no more treatment effect remains from therapy), the patient is rechecked to ensure that treatment does not need to be restarted.

Monitoring strategy

For all phases, there are several choices to be made in devising a good monitoring strategy: whether to monitor at all, the choice of measurement(s), the choice of target range, the choice of measurement interval and who should monitor.

Which measurement?

The more appropriate the measurement we choose the better we can guide therapy. There will often be a variety of possible monitoring tests, and there are advantages to choosing one main measurement (or a composite measure of several) to guide changes in management. The criteria for the choice of measurement include:

- Is it a good predictor of clinically relevant outcomes? Most monitoring measurements are surrogate markers (see below) for patient-relevant outcomes.[109]
- Can it detect changes in risk rapidly enough? Risk predictors will vary in their responsiveness to the beneficial impact of treatment, with a good monitoring measurement providing an early indication of risk change.
- Is the random variability acceptable, or can it be made acceptable by repeated measurements?
- Is it sufficiently affordable, accessible and acceptable to patients?

Surrogate measures

These are more easily measured substitutes for the patient outcomes that would be preferable, were they available. They can be proximal or distal.

Proximal targets, such as drug concentrations, have the advantage of being directly related, and often rapidly responsive to, changing therapy.

Distal targets, such as the clinical outcomes we aim to prevent, are the more important outcomes, but a perceptible response may involve a considerable time lag.

For example, for osteoporosis, monitoring measurements could include (from proximal to distal): patient adherence (e.g., through pill counts), drug concentrations, markers of bone turnover, bone mineral density (BMD), asymptomatic fractures (through spinal X-ray or bone scans), and finally symptomatic fractures. The choice involves a fundamental tradeoff between relevance (criterion 1) and rapid feedback (criterion 2). Figure 7.2 illustrates these trade-offs for some osteoporosis measures, for the two pathways of drug treatment and exercise.

This fundamental trade-off usually suggests intermediate measures as the appropriate compromise, which might be summarised as 'the most relevant measure that can be assessed reasonably soon'.

To complicate this trade-off, there may be the additional tradeoffs of variability and cost. A relative stable measurement with little day-to-day variation

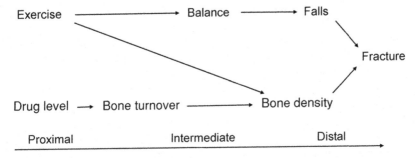

Figure 7.2 Trade-off between early detection of response and predictive: early changes (drug concentration or bone turnover markers) may be helpful to monitor response, but may be less predictive than late markers, though the final outcome may depend on several factors and pathways. From Glasziou et al.[89]

but with short-term (days to weeks) response to therapy would be ideal for outpatient adjustment of therapy.

In the monitoring of hypothyroidism, blood level of TSH is suitable, though out-of-range results may need to be supplemented with T3 and/or T4.

Glycosylated haemoglobin (HbA1c) is used for monitoring diabetes mellitus. The natural turnover of red blood cells (with about a 3-month life cycle) means that the measurement is relatively stable, reflects blood glucose control over a clinically useful length or time, and is a reasonably precise predictor of clinical outcome. However, HbA1c is only one of several proximal risk factors (others being blood pressure, cholesterol, smoking etc.) for the more distal changes of atherosclerosis and cardiovascular events.

Setting more than one target

Sometimes treatment decisions depend on the impact of treatment on a risk factor (a proximal measure) and the longer-term effect of treatment on the target condition (a distal measure).

For example, in normal-tension glaucoma, we monitor intra-ocular pressure (IOP) with the goal of reducing it by one third.[110] Less frequently we monitor visual fields, which only change slowly; therefore, real changes ('signal') are difficult to differentiate from the background 'noise' of this subjective test unless sufficient time has elapsed between monitoring measurements.

Measuring benefits and harms

The ideal target and action thresholds (see Figure 7.1) involve a trade-off between the potential benefits and adverse effects of different levels of treatment.

If these benefits and adverse effects are similar across all patients, then a single set of initiation and target thresholds is reasonable,

For example, monitoring warfarin for atrial fibrillation, a single target threshold of an INR (InterNational Ratio) of about 2.5 ± 0.5 (depending on different recommendations) is usual.

However, if the potential benefits are very different, then the initiation threshold, target (and action thresholds) need to be stratified or even individualised.

For example, with cholesterol reduction, target blood cholesterol levels are now appropriately different in primary versus secondary prevention.[111]

In these examples, the potential benefits and harms are the same across all patients (that is, as can be found from randomised trials). However, if possible, they should be refined by data collected from the individual patient, such as adverse effects.

Choosing the monitoring interval

The different phases require different monitoring interval (see Table 7.1). It is shortest for the pre-treatment phase, longest for the maintenance phase, and intermediate for the other three phases.

Pre-treatment

Even though the pre-treatment initiation phase requires the shortest measurements, these need to be far enough apart to allow for any short-term variability between days as well as within days.

For example, the multiple readings of a 24-hour blood pressure monitoring gives an accurate picture over a full day, but fails to capture the considerable day-to-day variability in some patients.

The optimal interval for monitoring during the initiation phase is usually the minimum time for each change of therapy to have maximal effect on the monitoring test. For drug treatment there are two considerations:

- *Pharmacokinetics:* How the drug disperses in the body? This requires at least 3–5 drug half-lives to reach near-steady-state concentration;
- *Pharmacodynamics:* What effect the drug has? This takes much longer to reach full physiological steady state.

A common mistake is to re-test too early. For example, the ACE-II inhibitor telmisartan has a half-life of 24 hours, and hence reaches a steady state in under a week, but it takes about 3 weeks (see Figure 7.3) for blood pressure reductions to stabilise.[112] Rechecking too early can thus lead to inappropriate adjustments. Anti-depressant treatment can take much longer than 2 weeks for the adverse effects to stabilise and the maximal clinical benefit to be achieved, and require the clinician and patient to 'hold steady' for a period before adjusting or switching treatment.

But conversely, one can re-test too late, thereby unduly prolonging the time taken to establish control.

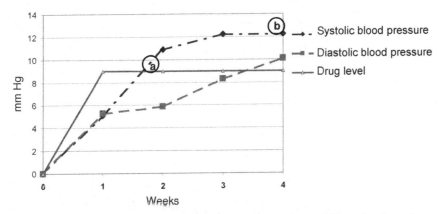

Figure 7.3 After initiating treatment: (a) drug concentration stabilises after 1 week, but (b) blood pressure takes 3–4 weeks to stabilise.

For example, for many of the common drugs used to treat glaucoma, the maximum clinical effect on intra-ocular pressure can often be achieved within hours – but is often only assessed at out-patient appointments that are seldom scheduled more frequently than monthly.[110]

For the maintenance phase, the optimal interval is a trade-off. Measuring too often risks detecting mostly false positive results and inappropriately adjusting treatment. Measuring too seldom risks allowing too many patients to drift out of control.

The rate of true positives will require data on how quickly patients may drift outside the control limits. As illustrated in Figure 7.4, this drift may be:

(a) *random*, where there is an accrual of changes in adherence, other drugs, diet, etc., which lead to some patients drifting lower and some higher (shaded tails in figure), but no change in the average value. This will lead to an increasing spread of the values of patients at re-measurement.

For example, prothrombin times for anticoagulated patients;

(b) *systematic*, where measurements get worse as, for example, the disease progresses.

For example, visual field loss in glaucoma.

Knowing the rate of both drifts enables us to predict the proportion of true positives, and hence the true positive to false positive ratio, which in turn provides a rational basis for setting the monitoring interval for stable patients.

Who should monitor?
Of course, monitoring is routinely part of the care a clinician provides. But patients can be very important monitors of their own disease, and

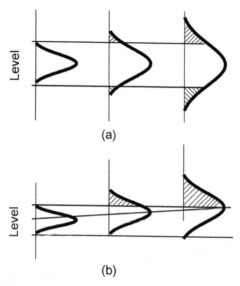

(a)

(b)

Figure 7.4 Drift from control may be (a) random in either direction, or (b) systematic increase (or decrease) over time. Shaded areas represent the tail of abnormal results.

self-monitoring is becoming more common. Their involvement might be at several levels.

- Simply reporting to the clinician (a source of monitoring information).

  For example, non-insulin dependent diabetic patients bring in diaries of their blood sugars to their primary care clinicians for planning any changes in medication.

  Similarly, home blood pressure monitoring provides data on which the clinician can decide future management.

- To improve adherence.

  For example, using pedometers to monitor physical activity;
  Or home blood glucose measurement for people with non-insulin dependent diabetics.

- An early warning system (reporting to medical care if the monitored measurement falls outside certain parameters).

  For example, patients with asthma using an 'asthma action plan' usually have several measures that they monitor: if these go past a certain stage of severity ('trigger actions'), then either they can summon medical help, or start some responsive action (such as starting steroids).

  Patients adjusting their own insulin doses to accommodate changes in energy expenditure and food eaten. This may have been the first published self-monitoring event: in 1975 a pregnant diabetic patient persuaded her doctor that home blood sugar measurements were feasible and preferable to her being hospitalised.[113]

Usually patients monitor their own disease for several of these categories. There can be benefits to both clinician workload and to patient's well being.

- Encouraging patients with asthma to self-monitor and adjust medication leads to reduced days of limited activity and improved quality of life.[114]
- Home blood pressure monitoring reduced mean blood pressure by 4.4mm Hg compared to standard blood pressure monitoring.[115] Though modest, this is similar to the impact of methods to improve adherence.[116]

However self-monitoring is not always welcome, nor cheaper.

- Randomised trials have shown that patients can manage anticoagulation with warfarin with home monitoring and self-adjusting therapy, with monitoring control equal to clinician monitoring, but at greater expense. And an important proportion, 45%, declined to participate.[117]

Self-monitoring should be based on an informed choice by the patient.

Common errors in monitoring

As we have seen, monitoring is a complex activity. Hence, slips and errors are likely. We will not attempt to catalogue all possible errors, but a few of the more common ones we have seen (or made ourselves!) include:

- Re-checking too soon. If we change therapy (e.g., change drug or change dose) it will take some time before equilibrium is reached again. For the drug plasma concentration to equilibrate takes a minimum of 5 half-lives. But pharmacodynamic equilibrium may take far longer. If we measure before this equilibrium is reached, we may be tempted to change course before the full effect is seen.
- Over-reacting to chance fluctuations. Most measurements of patients are far more variable than we perceive them to be. Hence we may be tempted to change therapy based on a chance fluctuation, which in turn leads to a real change, and a need to change therapy again. So a good rule of thumb is to check again before you change, unless the fluctuation is extreme.
- Over-adjusting therapy. We may also be tempted to make a substantial adjustment to make sure we achieve control again. However, in doing so we may overshoot the mark, and again get into a vicious cycle of adjustments. This appears common in warfarin monitoring, though is less of a problem in 'one-sided' targets such as blood pressure or cholesterol monitoring.

Common monitoring tests

See Table 7.2 for finding values to monitor different chronic diseases.

Table 7.2 Finding values to monitor different chronic diseases.

Disease	Value to monitor
NIDDM	HbA1c BSL or urine
Asthma	Symptoms (triggering need for PEFR measures)
Osteoarthritis	Visual analogue pain chart
Hypertension	BP
Depression	Beck questionnaire
Hypo-/hyperthyroid	Pulse and TSH (with T3 or T as needed).
Obesity	Weight or waist circumference
Heart Failure	Weight (or perhaps B-natriuretic peptide)
Parkinson's	Timed up-and-go test
Dementia	MMSE or clockface + 3-item recall
COAD/COPD	PF symptoms
Ischaemic Heart Disease	Walking distance
Periphereal vascular disease	Walking distance
Anticoagulation	INR of prothrombin time
Glaucoma	Intra-ocular pressure and visual fields
Skin lesions	Polaroid camera
Headaches	Frequency diary

Discussion

The principles of monitoring are not well taught to clinicians, despite being such a common activity in clinical practice. Chronic care could potentially be improved (and often at reduced costs) if for each chronic disease we:

- determined whether and how monitoring was necessary;
- set explicit monitoring ranges and provided appropriate graphical representations that aided decision making;
- recognised the need for different optimal intervals for different phases;
- better understood when and how to adjust therapy to avoid the increases in variability caused by over-adjustment.

There is a need for both better understanding of these principles for those working in chronic care, and system improvements including use of appropriate decision aids that have been shown to improve monitoring care.

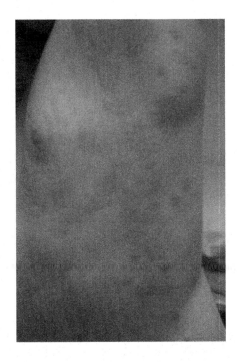

Figure 5.4 Clinical presentation of Pityriasis rosacea (Photo: Dr Michael Freeman, Gold Coast, Australia)

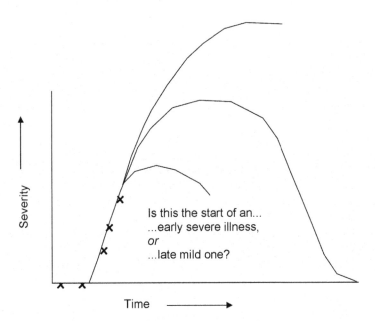

Severity

Is this the start of an...
...early severe illness,
or
...late mild one?

Time

Figure 5.5 The variability in the course of *Pityriasis rosacea*.

CHAPTER 8

Screening for disease, health promotion and disease prevention

We have seen how diseases have a natural history. For many diseases, there is a time when the disease is detectable but before symptoms become manifest. Detecting the disease and intervening in these early stages can sometimes reduce the impact of the disease (*'Disease screening'*, also called *'Early detection'*, all part of *secondary prevention*), but also has some important downsides such as over-detection and the anxiety of false positives.

We can also reduce the risk of death and morbidity by reducing the exposure to risk factors for disease before the process even starts *'Health promotion'*, or by providing interventions that prevent the disease from ever manifesting (*'Disease prevention'*). These are both *primary prevention.*

Primary prevention

This includes activities that are either general (such as life-style improvements) or specific (such as vaccinations against one disease, or using anticoagulation to prevent deep venous thrombosis during surgery).

Primary prevention aims to prevent a disease ever occurring, or at least reducing the chances of it happening.

Health promotion and prevention activities can act through reducing the exposure of individuals to the risk factors of disease or by acting to change the environment in which they live. It can be difficult to change the behaviour and the exposure of individuals without also changing the environment in which they live. Medical practitioners primarily work with individuals, but they also have a responsibility to advocate for a healthy environment for their patients (Figures 8.1 and 8.2 and Table 8.1).

When we think about the leading causes of death and disability, we usually think about diseases such as ischaemic heart disease and lung cancer. However, these diseases are just the end-manifestation of the disease process. Often they are the result of exposure to environmental or lifestyle factors. It is helpful to think of the most important causes of death in the developed world (Box 8.1).

Reducing the exposure of the population to these risk factors can help reduce the burden of disease and disability in a population. Many of the strategies for

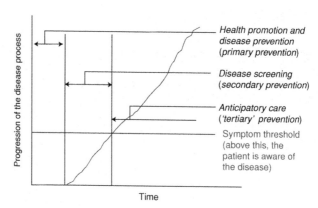

Figure 8.1 The potential to intervene to minimise the effects of disease.

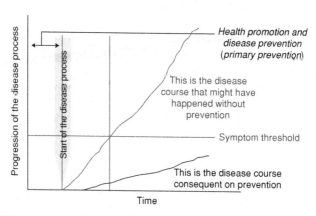

Figure 8.2 Primary prevention.

Table 8.1 Health promotion, disease prevention, screening and early detection.

Activity	What it does	Examples
Health promotion	Interventions that generally improve the health of everyone – without reference to any disease	Exercise, stopping smoking, eating well
Disease prevention	Pre-emptively acting before a specific disease is manifest	Vaccination, seatbelts, cycle helmets
Disease screening (also called early detection or secondary prevention)	Looking for signs of disease before they are manifest. 'A stitch in time...'	Mammography, measuring blood pressure, cervical screening
Anticipatory care (also called 'tertiary' prevention)	Looking for, and anticipating complications of a disease that is already diagnosed	Diabetes, heart failure, asthma (almost every chronic disease!)

It may be helpful to try to picture these different processes.

Box 8.1 The 10 Leading Risk Factors For Death In the Developed World[118]

- Tobacco use
- Inadequate or excessive nutrition (dietary habits)
- Inadequate aerobic exercise
- Excessive alcohol consumption
- Lack of immunisation against microbial agents
- Exposure to poisons and toxins
- Firearms
- Risky sexual behaviours
- Motor vehicle trauma
- Use of illicit drugs

health promotion can be implemented across an entire population, outside the context of medical consultations. For example, restricting cigarette smoking in public places reduces the exposure of the entire population to tobacco smoke, *and* discourages smokers from smoking.

Health promotion can also occur alongside the delivery of medical services.

Doing more harm than good

It is easy to forget that health promotion and disease prevention can do harm. Often the harm is minimal – representing no more than inconvenience, spending time and modest cost (see Figure 8.3).

So it is true that it is generally better to prevent diseases than to treat them once they have occurred. Also, there is little harm in changing the way people behave, so that they automatically become healthier. This usually involves dietary changes (eating a wide variety of fruit and vegetable, less meat

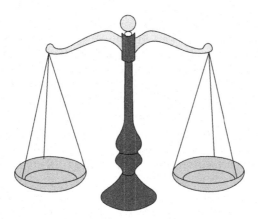

Figure 8.3 Scales: balancing good against harm.

Table 8.2 Examples of negative outcomes from health promotion.

Intervention (the primary prevention)	Unexpected negative outcome
Attempts to reduce alcohol problems in Poland by introduction of a policy to restrict alcohol purchases	The population reacting to the threat of shortages by hoarding vodka. People who had never drunk alcohol started drinking; illegal distillation increased[121]
An advertising campaign designed to shock people into avoiding sunlight in tropical Queensland, Australia, which showed graphic pictures of skin cancer operations	People worried about pigmented naevi visited the doctor in huge numbers; excision rates increased several-fold with no increase in melanomas detected[122]
Legislation for compulsory wearing of helmets while using a bicycle, to reduce head injuries	Fewer people cycling[123]

and saturated fat and more fish); not smoking; a modest alcohol consumption; vigorous weight bearing exercise several times a week; and avoiding sunlight.

However there can be harms. Many people loathe exercising, and would even trade some of their health to avoid it. Avoiding sunlight means losing some benefits (feeling better is one), some of which are health benefits (less depression) in favour of the risk of skin cancer.[119] Some people have been very critical of what is seen as a puritanical approach to making the majority of the population feel guilty about the way they live.[120] And there have been isolated instances in which public health messages have had unexpected and perverse outcomes (see Table 8.2).

Secondary prevention

These activities reduce the impact of a disease by intervening after the disease process has started, but before the disease starts to impact on the patient – specifically before the person (not yet a patient!) has noticed anything (Figure 8.4).

Examples include activities that involve the early detection of a disease, such as screening and contact tracing. For example:
- The treatment of hypertension and hypercholesterolaemia is secondary prevention for the development of ischaemic heart disease.
- Screening for the pre-cursors of cervical cancer (CIN changes) of the cervix is also secondary prevention.
- (Interventions that reduce the impact of a disease or injury *if* it occurs, such as enforcing the usage of seat belts, can be thought of as either primary *or* secondary prevention).

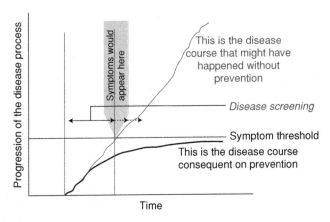

Figure 8.4 Secondary prevention.

Screening for disease

Screening for disease and intervening at an early stage in the disease process would seem to be an effective method for significantly reducing the potential harm from disease. There are certainly diseases where this is the case. It is not true, however, that screening always results in benefits

This example (see Figure 8.5) compares the pre-test probability (that is, the chance before the tests) of a woman having breast cancer plotted against the post-test probability for a standard work-up for breast cancer. As expected, the probability of negative tests hugely reduces the probability of having breast cancer, although the positive tests make only a slight improvement. However, the main point of interest is how the pre-test probability changes the chances of having a positive test.

Imagine a woman of about 70 years with symptoms of a breast lump. The chance that this is cancer is about 50% in that age group, in other words the pre-test probability is 0.5. Reading off the results of a positive test increase the chance that she has breast cancer to 0.75 (75%), but of a negative test to about 0.01 (1%). (See Chapter 4 on Diagnosis and Figures 4.6 and 4.7.)

Now imagine a woman coming for screening at the age of 55. Screening implies she has no symptoms relating to her breast: she has noticed no lumps, discomfort or nipple discharge. The chance she has breast cancer is very low: certainly less than 1%. One cannot even read off the graph because a positive test would still be so very low.

Screening tests are used quite differently from diagnostic tests. It is very important for screening programmes to not miss the diseases that are present. So they will use tests that are more sensitive and less specific than those used to diagnose disease. For example,

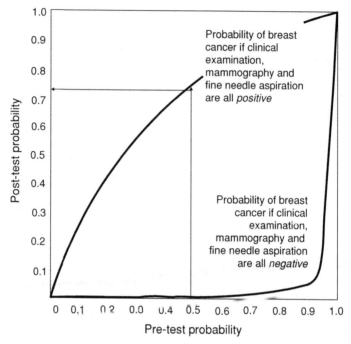

Figure 8.5 Comparison of the pre- and post-test probabilities of breast cancer after standard test 'work-up'.[124]

screening mammograms are used to detect any suspicious lesion – not to determine if a lesion is truly a breast cancer or not.

When we combine a test with a poor specificity with the low pre-test probability of disease in a screening population, the test will inevitably have a poor positive predictive value, that is, the probability the person has the disease is the screening test is positive.

For screening mammograms, the positive predictive value is about 10%. For the blood test used in Down syndrome in antenatal screening it is about 3%.

This raises concerns with screening tests. They have the ability to upset and frighten people like any other test. Because people undergoing screening tests have no illness, even greater care must be taken not to cause harm – especially psychological harm – when communicating results.

'...and so the lesion that was seen on the mammogram does not necessarily mean you have cancer of the breast. In fact the chance it is cancer is only about 10%...'

Box 8.2 Checklist to Decide if Screening is Worthwhile[125]

Preliminary or developers criteria
- Is the disease important?
- Is there an effective test?
- Is there effective treatment?
- Is the test affordable and acceptable?

User criteria
- Is the effective treatment *more* effective at an early stage?
- Do benefits outweigh harms?
- Is the test routinely available?

It is probably better that people understand the odds of a positive (and of a negative) screening test finally yielding a true positive *before* they embark on it. This is especially true of tests around which there is a lot of controversy, such as a PSA (prostate specific antigen) for prostate cancer screening.

'... And we can easily do the test. But remember that even if the test is positive, for someone in your age group, the chances of a needle biopsy subsequently finding prostate cancer would be only 1 in 20...'

What screening tests should we use?

How are we to decide what is worth screening for? The WHO has a checklist of important characteristics to check. We have separated this into preliminary or developers criteria, relevant to those planning whether a screening programme is even worth evaluating, and user criteria (see Box 8.2).[125] For the clinician, we only need to pay attention to the user criteria; that is, whether the screening programme has been rigorously evaluated and shown to be sufficiently effective for the benefits to outweigh harms.[126]

Let us see how some tests match up (see Table 8.3).

One has to therefore decide a balancing act: do the benefits outweigh the harms of screening? This has to be undertaken by setting out the harms and benefits in a way that enables them to be visualised (see Figure 8.6).

A test such as PSA performs poorly. More prostate cancers will be missed than discovered. (People who engage in screening yet whose cancers are missed feel especially cheated.) Moreover, the screening process itself can harm people. A large proportion of men who have a PSA test will need a follow-up biopsy (about 15%). Of the men who have a biopsy, about 2% will have a haemorrhage or infection severe enough to require a hospital admission. This means that out of the 100,000 men screened, 2,100 men who were otherwise healthy will be admitted to hospital as a result of having the screening test. Of the other 10,500 who needed a biopsy and who turned out not to have prostate cancer, there is the psychological stress of the positive screen result and subsequent investigation of the biopsy.

Table 8.3 Some possible screening tests and how they match up to the checklist.

Check-list question	Cervical cancer	Prostate cancer	Stroke, IHD	Phenyl-ketonuria	Lung cancer
Preliminary criteria					
Is the disease important?	√	√	√√√	√√√(Devastating, if rare)	√√√
Is there an effective test?	Pap smear	PSA ± digital exam	Blood pressure measurement	Heel prick of newborn	CXR
Is the test affordable and acceptable?	√	√	√√√	√√√√	√√√
Is there effective treatment	√√√	√?	√√√	√√√	X
User criteria					
Is the effective treatment *more* effective at an early stage?	√√	?	√√√	√√√	X
Do benefits outweigh harms?	Yes	?	Yes	Yes	No
Is the test routinely available?	Yes	No	Yes	Yes	No

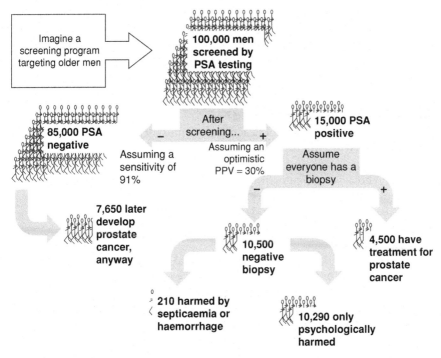

Figure 8.6 Visualising the benefits and harms from screening with a PSA (prostate specific antigen) blood test for prostate cancer (adapted from Hirst).[127]

Also, it is not clear which men who are diagnosed with prostate cancer after their biopsy are better off as a result of their diagnosis: we know that many men with prostate cancer (in fact the great proportion) do not die from the disease. But at present, we cannot predict for any individual whether they will benefit from treatment or not. It remains uncertain which sub-groups of prostate cancer are improved by radical prostatectomy. However, we know that most men are damaged by the treatment (90% are rendered impotent; and 20% suffer either faecal or urinary incontinence).

There are many individual diseases that can be diagnosed but which never cause any harm – patients might die *with* the disease rather than *from* them, so-called 'indolent' (lazy) tumours. Of course the ideal is to derive a screening test that distinguishes the indolent disease from the aggressive one. For many diseases this is not yet possible.

The poor performance of screening tests is best thought of in terms of false negative and false positives. It is a very important principle that false positives are more common in situations in which the disease rate is rare. This is part of Bayes' theorem (which explains how the usefulness of a test is dependent on the frequency of the disease being sought; see the previous Chapter on Diagnosis).

The issue does not stop there. The benefits outweigh harms for an increasing number of different screening possibilities. How do we decide which to do? The spectrum of possible preventive activities need to be ranked in terms of best benefits for each, so that they can be tackled in a rational manner.

When should screening be used?

Having decided to use a screening activity, we must decide what groups to use it for. Not everyone will benefit.

Men get breast cancer at such a low rate (1% of women) that this renders screening men for breast cancer unnecessary.

- Age groupings are less obvious.

Cervical cancer is associated with past sexual activity. The precursors to cancer develop over the next few years. So it is only necessary to screen women after a time interval from the start of sexual activity. Similarly the development of cervical cancer is slow enough to render screening for it unnecessary after the age of about 70 years of age (when the chance of being exposed to risk is much lower too).

- Other risk factors may be important.

We treat blood pressure earlier (that is, look for increased blood pressure earlier, and even treat at lower levels) when there are associated risks such as smoking or diabetes.

Tertiary prevention

These activities reduce the further risk of death and disability once a disease has become evident (Figure 8.7).

This is the other end of the spectrum. Here the focus is on prevention of the complications of a disease, and is usually the dominant component of chronic care (see Chapter 7 on Monitoring).

- In managing people with type 2 non-insulin-dependent diabetes mellitus, clinicians spend a lot of time trying to minimise the onset of complications such as diabetic retinopathy (by screening for it ophthalmologically), or careful foot inspection (to screen for early diabetic neuropathy), as well as encouraging tight glucose control.
- Heart failure involves checking for decompensation, checking adherence to drugs, checking the drugs are not disturbing the electrolytes and minimising any further progression of the cardiovascular disease (smoking, diet and exercise).

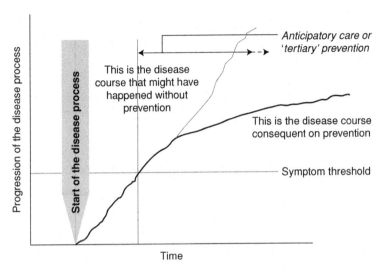

Figure 8.7 Tertiary prevention.

Incorporating health promotion, prevention and screening into the medical consultation

Incorporating disease prevention activities into medical consultations involves making three types of decisions:

• Which disorders to target
• Which sub-groups of the population to target
• Which interventions to use

Targeting interventions at persons who are at high risk of disease can allow the most benefit to be gained by those at the greatest risk. However, when a disease is common, it may be worth targeting even people at moderate risk who can gain from health promotion and preventive activities. Reducing the risk for a large number of people at moderate risk can result in greater overall benefits than targeting a small number of patients at high risk. This is the 'population strategy' advocated by Geoffrey Rose. He demonstrated that even a small shift in the whole population's distribution of total cholesterol levels resulted in a greater reduction in ischaemic heart disease mortality than in a larger reduction in total cholesterol levels in only those at high risk (see Table 8.4 and Figure 8.8).[128] But others question this paradigm. For example, modelling with ischemic heart disease suggests more than 70% of the fall in population mortality in the USA can be attributed to better initial treatment of myocardial infarction and improvements in tertiary prevention.[129]

As can be seen, deaths from cholesterol (curve 2) are related to its levels distributed in the population (curve 1) (see Figure 8.8). Using a targeted approach to prevention (that is, concentrating on high risk people) results in

Table 8.4 The effect of different approaches to prevention of deaths from cholesterol (see text). Data modified after Rose.[128]

		Total serum cholesterol (mmol/L)								
		< 4	4–4.5	4.5–5	5–5.5	5.5–6	6–6.5	6.5–7	7–7.5	> 7.5
Percentage (%)	Distribution of cholesterol level in the population	9	13	18	22	16	11	6	3	2
	Distribution of deaths attributable to high cholesterol effect	0	4	8	17	22	19	13	9	8
	Distribution of deaths after high-risk approach to cholesterol lowering	0	4	8	21.5	26.2	22.5	—	—	—
	Distribution of deaths after population approach to cholesterol lowering	0	5.6	3.7	12.3	15.2	10.4	6.5	6.0	—

This may be easier to visualise graphically (see Figure 8.8).

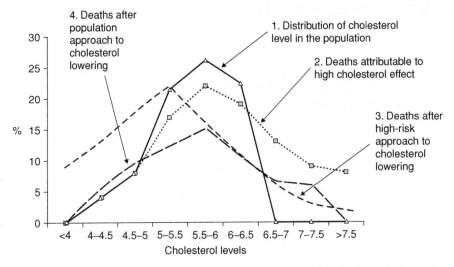

Figure 8.8 The effect of different approaches to prevention of deaths from cholesterol (see text). Data modified after Rose.[128]

fewer deaths (curve 3), especially at the high-risk end. However, a population approach (curve 4), results in even fewer deaths overall (imagine the area under the curve) even though relatively more die at the very high-risk end. Is a population approach always preferable? Not always.

The population strategy will be preferable when:

- the target disorder is common and a large proportion of the population is exposed to risk factors for the target disorder;
- where the risk of disease rises continuously with exposure to the risk factor (as occurs with blood pressure and cholesterol levels); and
- where it is easier or cheaper to apply an intervention to an entire population than to find and direct the interventions to individuals at high risk of the target disorder.

Effective health promotion activities, such as encouraging healthy eating and increased physical activity, are usually accompanied by so little disadvantage that they are worth conducting whenever possible.

What is more contentious is whether we should use drugs for whole populations at risk. For example some have advocated the 'poly-pill' (a cocktail of preventive drugs designed to lower cholesterol, lower blood pressure and replace possible folate deficiency) for the whole population over a certain age.[130]

A targeted approach is preferable when:

- exposure to the risk factor is more limited within the population;
- where the susceptibility following exposure to the risk factor is limited, or where there is a threshold effect;

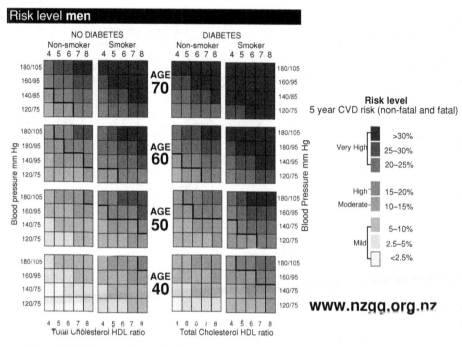

Figure 8.9 Chart used for calculating risk of cardiovascular disease for designing preventive activities for men (a different chart exists for women).

- where it is easier or cheaper to identify persons at high risk; and
- the intervention is difficult to comply with or carries a significant risk of side effects.

Currently we use targeted approaches more as clinicians (while epidemiologists and public health physicians focus more on population approaches). In addition, the two approaches often come together, where clinicians can talk about health promotion and disease prevention as part of the consultation when the patient has come for some other reasons to the doctor.[21] This is a time of increased susceptibility to messages about changing lifestyle.

These cardiovascular charts (see Figure 8.9) compare the relative impact of different risk factors on the baseline risk for a cardiovascular 'event' (myocardial infarction or cerebrovascular accident). Thus it can be seen that we elect to treat people with a risk of 15–20% in the next 5 years, then we will wait to treat non-smoking men without diabetes in their 70s until their systolic blood pressure reaches 140, while even if they are normotensive, but smoking and diabetic, it is worth treating with antihypertensives.

Remembering to provide prevention

It is important to ensure that disease prevention and health promotion are not forgotten in the time-pressured consultation. Patients are usually focussed on

Table 8.5 The exceptional opportunity in every consultation: prevention as one of the four central duties of the doctor.[21]

Why has the patient come? (Addressing the patient's concerns)	A	B	*Health promotion, disease prevention*
Other health risks from pre-existing illnesses	C	D	Issues of access to future care (follow-up arrangements, self-care etc.)

the reason fro their visit. How can the clinician remember to check on at least some of the possible preventive activities? One way is to mark off one time in the consultation for this. We saw in Chapter 2 (Communication) how prevention was promoted into a model as one of four main sets of 'tasks of the consultation' (Table 8.5).[21] The clinician is encouraged to check that some prevention is thought about at every visit – the 'exceptional potential in every consultation'.

This was manifest as a simple reminder to help general practitioners remember to at least consider health promotion and disease prevention as a part of every consultation.

The promoters of this approach considered that doctors should have this table pinned to the wall behind the patient, within eyesight.

'… Now we have sorted that out, I just wanted to check on some things to do with your health. I don't see a blood pressure recording here in your record. When was the last time we measured that … ?'

'… Just remind me: you aren't a smoker are you?'

When it comes to deciding which preventive activity to do first, we need some idea of which preventive activities give the most health benefit for effort, and according to the patient's own priorities. This might be a good time to re-read the section at the end of Chapter 2 on Communication.

CHAPTER 9
Endpiece

What next? We hope you find some of this book helpful in looking after patients, or teaching medical students or young doctors to do so.

Although we have tried to minimise them, we recognise that there are probably many shortcomings, and sub-optimal examples. If you can think of ways of improving the book, please do not hesitate to contact us. Our e-mail addresses are below, and we would love to hear from you if you have any comments to provide. We might even incorporate improvements (suitably acknowledged of course) in a future edition.

However, in addition we have some teaching slides made up of the contents here that you can access at the following web site:

http://www.bond.edu.au/ClinicalThinking/

Finally, we hope this book stimulates you also to find the evidence to add that ingredient to good patient care. We also think that this book contributes to making patient care, that most satisfying responsibility, even more fun!

Chris Del Mar
CDelMar@bond.edu.au

Jenny Doust
J.Doust@uq.edu.au

Paul Glasziou
paul.glasziou@dphpc.ox.ac.uk

References

1 Sackett DL, Straus SE, Richardson WS, Rosenberg W, Haynes RB. Evidence-based medicine. How to practice and teach EBM. 2nd ed. Edinburgh: Churchill Livingstone, 2000.

2 Dreyfus HL, Dreyfus SE. Mind over machine: the power of human intuition and expertise in the era of the computer. Oxford: Blackwell, 1986.

3 Norman G. Research in clinical reasoning: past history and current trends. Med Educ 2005;39:418–27.

4 Greenhalgh T. Uneasy bedfellows: reconciling intuition and evidence based practice. YoungMinds Magazine 2002;59:23–27.

5 Eddy D. Medicine, money and mathematics. Bull Am Coll Surg 1992;77:48.

6 Klein G. Sources of power: how people make decisions. Cambridge: MIT Press, 1999.

7 Gigerenzer G. Simple heuristics that make us smart. Oxford: Oxford University Press, 2000.

8 Hunink M, Glasziou P. Decision making in health and medicine: integrating evidence and values. Cambridge: Cambridge University Press, 2001.

9 Hammond J, Keeney R, Raiffa H. Smart choices: a practical guide to making better decisions. New York: Broadway Books, 1998.

10 von Neumann J, Morgenstern O. Theory of games and economic behavior. Princeton: Princeton University Press, 1944.

11 Karras DJ, Ong S, Moran GJ, Nakase J, Kuehnert MJ, Jarvis WR, et al. Antibiotic use for emergency department patients with acute diarrhea: prescribing practices, patient expectations, and patient satisfaction. Ann Emerg Med 2003;42:835–42.

12 Mehta SR, Cannon CP, Fox KA, Wallentin L, Boden WE, Spacek R, et al. Routine vs selective invasive strategies in patients with acute coronary syndromes: a collaborative meta-analysis of randomized trials. JAMA 2005;293:2908–17.

13 NHMRC. Communicating with patients. Advice for medical practitioners. Canberra: NHMRC working party, 2004.

14 Stewart MA. Effective physician–patient communication and health outcomes: a review. Can Med Assoc J 1995;152:1423–33.

15 Hampton JR, Harrison MJ, Mitchell JR, Prichard JS, Seymour C. Relative contributions of history-taking, physical examination, and laboratory investigation to diagnosis and management of medical outpatients. BMJ 1975;2:486–9.

16 Hoffbrand BI. Away with the system review: a plea for parsimony. BMJ 1989; 298:817–9.

17 Byrne PF, Long BEL. Doctors talking to patients. London: HMSO. Royal College of General Practitoners, 1976.

18 Beckman HB, Frankel RM. The effect of physician behavior on the collection of data. Ann Intern Med 1984;101:692–6.

19 Lang F, Floyd MR, Beine KL, Buck P. Sequenced questioning to elicit the patient's perspective on illness: effects on information disclosure, patient satisfaction, and time expenditure. Fam Med 2002;34:325–30.

20 Pendleton DA, Schofield TPC, Tate PHL, Havelock PB. The consultation; an approach to learning and teaching. Oxford: Oxford University Press, 1984.

21 Stott NCH, Davis RH. The exceptional potential in each primary care consultation. J Roy Col Gen Pract 1979;29:201–205.

22 Botelho RJ. A negotiation model for the doctor-patient relationship. Fam Practice 1992;9:210–18.

23 Langewitz W, Denz M, Keller A, Kiss A, Ruttimann S, Wossmer B. Spontaneous talking time at start of consultation in outpatient clinic: cohort study. BMJ 2002;325:682–3.

24 Del Mar CB. Communicating well in general practice. Med J Aust 1994;160:367–70.

25 Kinmonth AL, Woodcock A, Griffin S, Spiegal N, Campbell MJ. Randomised controlled trial of patient centred care of diabetes in general practice: impact on current wellbeing and future disease risk. The Diabetes Care From Diagnosis Research Team. BMJ 1998;317:1202–8.

26 Feinstein RE, Feinstein MS. Psychotherapy for health and lifestyle change. J Clin Psychol 2001;57:1263–75.

27 Neighbour R. Checkpoint 4 (safety-netting) – predicting skills. The inner consultation. Oxford: Radcliffe Publishing, 2005:225–232.

28 Levinson W. Physician-patient communication. A key to malpractice prevention [editorial]. JAMA 1994;272:1619–20.

29 Del Mar C, Henderson M. Communicating bad news to patients and relatives. In: Sanders MR, Mitchell C, Byrne GJA, editors. Medical consultation skills: behavioural and interpersonal dimensions of health care. Melbourne: Addison-Wesley, 1997:103–17.

30 Skene L, Smallwood R. What should doctors tell patients? Med J Aust 1993;159:367–8.

31 Holland JC, Geary N, Marchini A, Tross S. An international survey of physician attitudes and practice in regard to revealing the diagnosis of cancer. Cancer Invest 1987;5:151–4.

32 Tayler M, Ogden J. Doctors' use of euphemisms and their impact on patients' beliefs about health: an experimental study of heart failure. Patient Educ Couns 2005;57:321–6.

33 Fallowfield L. Giving sad and bad news. Lancet 1993;341:476–478.

34 O'Dowd TC. Five years of heartsink patients in general practice. BMJ 1988;297:528–30.

35 Law MR, Wald NJ. Risk factor thresholds: their existence under scrutiny. BMJ 2002;324:1570–6.

36 Ryle JA. The natural history of disease. 2nd ed. London: Oxford University Press, 1948.

37 Faergeman O. The atherosclerosis epidemic: methodology, nosology, and clinical practice. Am J Cardiol 2001;88:4E–7E.

38 Anonymous. Coding matters. Newletter of the National Centre for Classification in Health (Australia), 2001:2.

39 Richards D, Toop L, Chambers S, Fletcher L. Response to antibiotics of women with symptoms of urinary tract infection but negative dipstick urine test results: double blind randomised controlled trial. BMJ 2005;331:143.

40 Norman GR, Coblentz CL, Brooks LR, Babcook CJ. Expertise in visual diagnosis: a review of the literature. Acad Med 1992;67:S78–83.

41 Elstein AS, Shulman LS, Sprafka SA. Medical problem solving: an analysis of clinical reasoning. Cambridge, Mass: Harvard University Press, 1978.

42 Barrows HS, Feltovich PJ. The clinical reasoning process. Med Educ 1987;21:86–91.

43 Coderre S, Mandin H, Harasym PH, Fick GH. Diagnostic reasoning strategies and diagnostic success. Med Educ 2003;37:695–703.

44 Williamson JW. Quality of current diagnostic performance: our most serious health care quality problem? [editorial]. Am J Med Qual 1994;9:145–48.

45 Green S, Price J. Complaints. Pulse 1998;63:67.

46 Vincent C, Neale G, Woloshynowych M. Adverse events in British hospitals: preliminary retrospective record review. BMJ 2001;322:517–9.

47 Bordage G. Why did I miss the diagnosis? Some cognitive explanations and educational implications. Acad Med 1999;74:S138–43.

48 Kassirer JP, Kopelman RI. Cognitive errors in diagnosis: instantiation, classification, and consequences. Am J Med 1989;86:433–41.

49 Goroll AH, Mulley AG, editors. Primary care medicine. Philadelphia: Lippincott, Williams and Wilkins, 2000.

50 Kahneman D, Slovic P, Tversky A, editors. Judgment under uncertainty: heuristics and biases. Cambridge: Cambridge University Press, 1982.

51 Elstein AS. Heuristics and biases: selected errors in clinical reasoning. Acad Med 1999;74:791–4.

52 Meador CK. A little book of doctors' rules. Philadelphia: Hanley and Belfus, 1992.

53 Richardson WS, Wilson MC. Textbook descriptions of disease–where's the beef? ACP J Club 2002;137:A11–2.

54 Friedman MH, Connell KJ, Olthoff AJ, Sinacore JM, Bordage G. Medical student errors in making a diagnosis. Acad Med 1998;73:S19–21.

55 Gruppen LD, Wolf FM, Billi JE. Information gathering and integration as sources of error in diagnostic decision making. Med Decis Making 1991;11:233–9.

56 Gruppen LD, Wisdom K, Anderson DS, Woolliscroft JO. An assessment of the impact of ambulatory care education of third-year medical students. Acad Med 1991;66:S55–7.

57 Lyman GH, Balducci L. Overestimation of test effects in clinical judgment. J Cancer Educ 1993;8:297–307.

58 Christensen-Szalanski JJ, Bushyhead JB. Physicians' misunderstanding of normal findings. Med Decis Making 1983;3:169–75.

59 Wolf FM, Gruppen LD, Billi JE. Differential diagnosis and the competing-hypotheses heuristic. A practical approach to judgment under uncertainty and Bayesian probability. JAMA 1985;253:2858–62.

60 Edwards W. Conservatism in human information processing. In: Kleinmuntz B, editor. Formal Representation of Human Judgment. New York: Wiley, 1968.

61 Bergus GR, Chapman GB, Gjerde C, Elstein AS. Clinical reasoning about new symptoms despite preexisting disease: sources of error and order effects. Fam Med 1995;27:314–20.

62 Chapman GB, Bergus GR, Elstein AS. Order of information affects clinical judgement. J Behav Decis Making 1996;9:201–11.

63 Kassirer JP, Kopelman RI. Learning clinical reasoning. Baltimore: Williams & Wilkins, 1991.

64 Asher R. Intracranial and extracranial computers. Middlesex Hospital Journal 1966.

65 Joseph GM, Patel VL. Domain knowledge and hypothesis generation in diagnostic reasoning. Med Decis Making 1990;10:31–46.

66 Lemieux M, Bordage G. Propositional versus structural semantic analyses of medical diagnostic thinking,. Cognitive Science 1992;16:185–204.

67 Murtagh J. Common problems: a safe diagnostic strategy. Aust Fam Physician 1990;19:733–40.

68 Murtagh J. General practice. 3rd ed. Melbourne: McGraw-Hill, 2003.

69 Balla JI, Biggs JB, Gibson M, Chang AM. The application of basic science concepts to clinical problem-solving. Med Educ 1990;24:137–47.

70 Banks E, Reeves G, Beral V, Bull D, Crossley B, Simmonds M, et al. Influence of personal characteristics of individual women on sensitivity and specificity of mammography in the Million Women Study: cohort study. BMJ 2004;329:477.

71 Irwig L. Report to the NBCC: Evidence relevant to guidelines for the diagnosis of symptomatic women. Sydney, 1996.

72 Sackett DL, Haynes RB, Guyatt GH, Tugwell P, editors. Clinical epidemiology: a basic science for clinical medicine. 2nd ed. Boston: Little, Brown and Company, 1991.

73 Hayward R. VOMIT (victims of modern imaging technology) – an acronym for our times. BMJ 2003;326:1273.

74 Kassirer JP. Teaching problem-solving – how are we doing? N Engl J Med 1995;332:1507–9.

75 Kassirer JP. Teaching clinical medicine by iterative hypothesis testing. Let's preach what we practice. N Engl J Med 1983;309:921–3.

76 Schmidt HG, Norman GR, Boshuizen HP. A cognitive perspective on medical expertise: theory and implication. Acad Med 1990;65:611–21.

77 Elstein AS, Schwartz A. Clinical reasoning in medicine. In: Higgs J, Jones M, editors. Clinical reasoning in the health professions. Oxford: Butterworth–Heinemann, 2002.

78 U.S. National Library of Medicine. http://www.ncbi.nl.nih.gov. In: PubMed, editor. 8600 Rockville Pike, Bethesda, MD 20894.

79 Cochrane Library. http://www3.interscience.wiley.com/cgi-bin/mrwhome/106568753/HOME.

80 Barton S, editor. Clinical evidence. A compendium of the best available evidence for effective health care. 7th ed. London: BMJ Group, 2005.

81 UpToDate. http://www.uptodate.com.

82 Glasziou PP, Del Mar CB, Hayem M, Sanders SL. Antibiotics for acute otitis media in children (Cochrane Review). Cochrane Database Syst Rev 2000;4.

83 Straus SE, Richardson WS, Rosenberg W, Haynes RB, Glasziou PP. Evidence-based medicine. How to practice and teach EBM. 3rd ed. Edinburgh: Churchill Livingstone, 2005.

84 Glasziou P, Del Mar C, Salisbury J. Evidence-based medicine workbook. Finding and applying the best research evidence to improve patient care. 1st ed. London: BMJ Books, 2003.

85 Damoiseaux RA, van Balen FA, Hoes AW, Verheij TJ, de Melker RA. Primary care based randomised, double blind trial of amoxicillin versus placebo for acute otitis media in children aged under 2 years. BMJ 2000;320:350–4.

86 Badenoch D, Heneghan C. Evidence-based medicine toolkit. London: BMJ Books, 2002.

87 Cates C. http://www.nntonline.net/ebm/newsletter/200210/200210.asp, 2005.

88 Sharland M, Kendall H, Yeates D, Randall A, Hughes G, Glasziou P, et al. Antibiotic prescribing in general practice and hospital admissions for peritonsillar abscess, mastoiditis, and rheumatic fever in children: time trend analysis. BMJ 2005;331:328–9.

89 Glasziou PP, Irwig L, Mant D. Monitoring in chronic disease: A rational approach. BMJ 2005;330:614–8.

90 Chen P, Tanasijevic MJ, Schoenenberger RA, Fiskio J, Kuperman GJ, Bates DW. A computer-based intervention for improving the appropriateness of antiepileptic drug level monitoring. Am J Clin Pathol 2003;119:432–8.

91 Ryan PJ, Gilbert M, Rose PE. Computer control of anticoagulant dose for therapeutic management. BMJ 1989;299:1207–9.

92 Gibson PG, Wlodarczyk J, Hensley MJ, Murree-Allen K, Olson LG, Saltos N. Using quality-control analysis of peak expiratory flow recordings to guide therapy for asthma. Ann Intern Med 1995;123:488–92.

93 Jannuzzi G, Cian P, Fattore C, Gatti G, Bartoli A, Monaco F, et al. A multicenter randomized controlled trial on the clinical impact of therapeutic drug monitoring in patients with newly diagnosed epilepsy. The Italian TDM Study Group in Epilepsy. Epilepsia 2000;41:222–30.

94 Rachmani R, Levi Z, Slavachevski I, Avin M, Ravid M. Teaching patients to monitor their risk factors retards the progression of vascular complications in high-risk patients with Type 2 diabetes mellitus – a randomized prospective study. Diabet Med 2002;19:385–92.

95 Robertson I, Phillips A, Mant D, Thorogood M, Fowler G, Fuller A, et al. Motivational effect of cholesterol measurement in general practice health checks. Br J Gen Pract 1992;42:469–72.

96 Yoos HL, Kitzman H, McMullen A, Henderson C, Sidora K. Symptom monitoring in childhood asthma: a randomized clinical trial comparing peak expiratory flow rate with symptom monitoring. Ann Allergy Asthma Immunol 2002;88:283–91.

97 Bland JM, Altman DG. Regression towards the mean. BMJ 1994;308:1499.

98 Dauber TR. The Framingham Study: The epidemiology of atherosclerotic disease. Cambridge, Mass: Harvard University Press, 1980.

99 Brueren MM, Petri H, van Weel C, van Ree JW. How many measurements are necessary in diagnosing mild to moderate hypertension? Fam Pract 1997;14:130–5.

100 Peyvandi F, Spreafico M, Siboni SM, Moia M, Mannucci PM. CYP2C9 genotypes and dose requirements during the induction phase of oral anticoagulant therapy. Clin Pharmacol Ther 2004;75:198–203.

101 Braithwaite RA, Dawling S, Montgomery SA. Prediction of steady-state plasma concentrations and individual dosage regimens of tricyclic antidepressants from a single test dose. Ther Drug Monit 1982;4:27–31.

102 Guyatt GH, Keller JL, Jaeschke R, Rosenbloom D, Adachi JD, Newhouse MT. The n-of-1 randomized controlled trial: clinical usefulness. Our three-year experience. Ann Intern Med 1990;112:293–9.

103 Irwig L, Glasziou P, Wilson A, Macaskill P. Estimating an individual's true cholesterol level and response to intervention. JAMA 1991;266:1678–85.

104 Aronson JK, Ferner RE. Joining the DoTS: new approach to classifying adverse drug reactions. BMJ 2003;327:1222–5.

105 Pirmohamed M, Ferner RE. Monitoring drug treatment. BMJ 2003;327:1179–81.

106 Boggs PB, Hayati F, Washburne WF, Wheeler DA. Using statistical process control charts for the continual improvement of asthma care. Jt Comm J Qual Improv 1999;25:163–81.

107 Sidwell A, Barclay M, Begg E, Moore G. Digoxin therapeutic drug monitoring: an audit and review. N Z Med J 2003;116:U708.

108 Bonnet C, Gagnayre R, d'Ivernois JF. Learning difficulties of diabetic patients: a survey of educators. Patient Educ Couns 1998;35:139–47.

109 Begg CB, Leung D. On the use of surrogate end points in randomized trials. J R Stat Soc [Ser A] 2000;163:15–28.

110 Irwig L. 'This added to my multiple myopia'. BMJ 2003;326:1336.

111 SIGN publication No 40. SIGN Lipids and the primary prevention of coronary heart disease. http://www.sign.ac.uk/guidelines/fulltext/40/index.html 1999.

112 Smith DH, Matzek KM, Kempthorne-Rawson J. Dose response and safety of telmisartan in patients with mild to moderate hypertension. J Clin Pharmacol 2000;40:1380–90.

113 Lowy C. Home glucose monitoring, who started it? BMJ 1998;316:1467.

114 Thoonen BP, Schermer TR, Van Den Boom G, Molema J, Folgering H, Akkermans RP, et al. Self-management of asthma in general practice, asthma control and quality of life: a randomised controlled trial. Thorax 2003;58:30–6.

115 Cappuccio FP, Kerry SM, Forbes L, Donald A. Blood pressure control by home monitoring: meta-analysis of randomised trials. BMJ 2004;329:145.

116 Schroeder K, Fahey T, Ebrahim S. How can we improve adherence to blood pressure-lowering medication in ambulatory care? Systematic review of randomized controlled trials. Arch Intern Med 2004;164:722–32.

117 Fitzmaurice DA, Murray ET, Gee KM, Allan TF, Hobbs FD. A randomised controlled trial of patient self-management of oral anticoagulation treatment compared with primary care management. J Clin Pathol 2002;55:845–9.

118 McGinnis JM, Foege WH. Actual causes of death in the United States. JAMA 1993;270:2207–12.

119 Ness AR, Frankel SJ, Gunnell DJ, Smith GD. Are we really dying for a tan? BMJ 1999;319:114–16.

120 Skrabanek P, McCormick J. Follies and fallacies in medicine. Glasgow: The Tarragon Press, 1989.

121 Smith R. Polish lessons on alcohol policy. BMJ 1982;284:98–101.

122 Del Mar CB, Green AC, Battistutta D. Do public media campaigns designed to increase skin cancer awareness result in increased skin excision rates? Aust NZ J Public Health 1997;21:751–3.

123 Wardlaw MJ. Three lessons for a better cycling future. BMJ 2000;321:1582–5.

124 NHMRC. Current best advice about familial aspects of breast cancer. Sydney, Australia: National Breast Cancer Centre, Genetic Testing Workgroup, 1996.

125 Wilson JM. Multiple screening. Lancet 1963;2:51–4.

126 Barratt A, Irwig L, Glasziou P, Cumming RG, Raffle A, Hicks N, et al. Users' guide to the medical literature: XVII. How to use guidelines and recommendations about screening. Evidence-Based Medicine Working Group. JAMA 1999;281:2029–34.

127 Hirst G, Ward J, Del Mar C. Screening for prostate cancer: the case against. Med J Aust 1996;164:285–8.

128 Rose G, Shipley M. Plasma cholesterol concentration and death from coronary heart disease: 10-year results of the Whitehall study. BMJ 1986;293:306–7.

129 Hunink MG, Goldman L, Tosteson AN, Mittleman MA, Goldman PA, Williams LW, et al. The recent decline in mortality from coronary heart disease, 1980–1990. The effect of secular trends in risk factors and treatment. JAMA 1997;277:535–42.
130 Wald NJ, Law MR. A strategy to reduce cardiovascular disease by more than 80%. BMJ 2003;326:1419.

Index

Page numbers in *italics* indicate figures; page numbers in **bold** indicate tables.

Lightning Source UK Ltd.
Milton Keynes UK
UKOW01f2309270917
309996UK00005B/129/P